The Hunchback in Hellenistic and Roman Art

Also Available From Bloomsbury

Hellenistic Tragedy, Agnieszka Kotlińska-Toma
Introduction to Greek Art, 2nd edition, Susan Woodford
The Trojan War in Ancient Art, Susan Woodford

The Hunchback in Hellenistic and Roman Art

Lisa Trentin

Bloomsbury Academic
An imprint of Bloomsbury Publishing Plc
B L O O M S B U R Y
LONDON • OXFORD • NEW YORK • NEW DELHI • SYDNEY

Bloomsbury Academic
An imprint of Bloomsbury Publishing Plc

50 Bedford Square
London
WC1B 3DP
UK

1385 Broadway
New York
NY 10018
USA

www.bloomsbury.com

BLOOMSBURY and the Diana logo are trademarks of Bloomsbury Publishing Plc

First published 2015
Paperback edition first published 2016

British Library Cataloguing-in-Publication Data
A catalogue record for this book is available from the British Library.

ISBN: HB: 978-1-78093-856-1
PB: 978-1-350-01914-0
ePDF: 978-1-78093-912-4
ePub: 978-1-78093-911-7

Library of Congress Cataloging-in-Publication Data
Trentin, Lisa, author.
The hunchback in Hellenistic and Roman art / Lisa Trentin.
pages cm
Based on the author's thesis (Ph. D.—University of Nottingham, 2007).
Includes bibliographical references and index.
ISBN 978-1-78093-856-1 (hardback)
1. Abnormalities, Human, in art. 2. Other (Philosophy) in art.
3. Art, Hellenistic. 4. Art, Roman. I. Title. N8236.P4T74 2015
759.6—dc23
2015009459

Typeset by RefineCatch Limited, Bungay, Suffolk

For mom and dad with love, always . . .

Contents

List of Illustrations

Preface

This book began life as a doctoral thesis written at the University of Nottingham between 2003 and 2007. The seeds for this project, however, were planted years earlier as an undergraduate student in Classical Archaeology at Wilfrid Laurier University. A senior seminar in 'Hellenistic Art and Architecture' introduced me to the 'other' side of the Classical ideal and my views on ancient art and the body beautiful were forever changed. What followed were several years of postgraduate work exploring representations of abnormality in the ancient Greco-Roman world: an MA dissertation at the University of Reading on 'Hermaphrodites in Roman Society and Sculpture' and a PhD thesis at the University of Nottingham on 'What's in a Hump? Re-presenting Deformity in Greco-Roman Art'. The first of these placed itself firmly within the wide and well-established gamut of research exploring the body of the hermaphrodite; the latter placed itself proudly at the forefront of new research exploring the body of the hunchback.

The figure of the hunchback has received relatively little scholarly attention, resulting in a significant gap in this field of research. The wealth of surviving evidence for the hunchback in both the literary and visual records is in itself sufficient motivation for further inquiry; however, no detailed study has yet been undertaken. My research seeks to put the figure of the hunchback back on the map, so to speak, by giving the hunchback the attention that it has been hitherto denied in the academy at large. My hope for this book extends beyond this: to provide a source of reference for future scholarly investigation that will continue to advance our knowledge of the hunchback, and more broadly, representations of the deformed and disabled Other in Classical antiquity.

Acknowledgements

This project is the result of years of research which formally began during my doctorate; I am grateful to the many people who helped see it to completion. Above all, I owe the greatest debt to my doctoral supervisor, Caroline Vout, who has been a true friend and mentor throughout my academic career. I thank too my PhD examiners, Catharine Edwards and Katarina Lorenz, for their recommendations in developing this project for publication. Although I have worked closely from the structure of my doctorate, all of the contents have been revisited and rewritten: two chapters of that original work have appeared in print elsewhere (Trentin 2009, 2011) and a new chapter has been added.

While turning this from thesis to book I worked in the Department of Archaeology and Classical Studies at my alma mater, Wilfrid Laurier University. Special thanks must go to Judith Fletcher, who has been endlessly generous with her time, intellect and encouragement over the past decade, first as my professor and then as my colleague. I am also grateful to have received generous funding from the Faculty of Arts to support the costs of reproducing the photographs in this book.

I wish also to thank Deborah Blake, Charlotte Loveridge, Anna MacDiarmid, Dhara Patel and Alice Reid, the Classics editorial team, past and present, at Bloomsbury Academic for their guidance and patience throughout, and the reviewers of my manuscript, Barbara Kellum and Jane Masséglia, for their generous feedback and judicious commentary. To Duncan Hill, who read multiple drafts of this work with great care and offered valuable suggestions for its improvement, and who, moreover, was always close by with words of comfort and cheer, you are truly a patient and treasured friend – thank you!

Last, but by no means least, I extend heartfelt thanks to my family and friends whose support and encouragement have known no bounds. Without you all, none of this would have been worthwhile.

Lisa Trentin
Toronto, 2014

Abbreviations

Ancient texts are cited in the notes according to the *Oxford Classical Dictionary* (fourth edition). All translations are from the Loeb Classical Library unless otherwise indicated. Modern sources repeatedly referenced in the chapters that follow are here listed. All other references are cited in full in the bibliography.

Bartman, *Miniature*	Bartman, E. (1992), *Ancient Sculptural Copies in Miniature*, Leiden: Brill.
Dasen, *Dwarfs*	Dasen, V. (1993), *Dwarfs in Ancient Egypt and Greece*, Oxford: Clarendon Press.
Garland, *Beholder*	Garland, R. (1995, 2010), *The Eye of the Beholder: Deformity and Disability in the Graeco-Roman World*, London: Bristol Classical Press.
Garmaise, *Dwarfs*	Garmaise, M. (1996), 'Studies in the Representation of Dwarfs in Hellenistic and Roman Art', PhD thesis, McMaster University.
Levi, *Lucky Hunchback*	Levi, D. (1941), 'The Evil Eye and the Lucky Hunchback', in R. Stillwell (ed.), *Antioch-on-the-Orontes*, vol. 3, Princeton: Princeton University Press.
Masséglia, *Body Language*	Masséglia, J. (2015), *Body Language in Hellenistic Art and Society*, Oxford: Oxford University Press.
Richter, *Grotesques*	Richter, G. M. A. (1913), 'Grotesques and the Mime', *American Journal of Archaeology* 17: 149–56.

Stevenson, *Pathological Grotesque*	Stevenson, W. E. (1975), 'The Pathological Grotesque Representations in Greek and Roman Art', PhD thesis, University of Pennsylvania.
Wace, *Grotesques*	Wace, A. J. B. (1903–04), 'Grotesques and the Evil Eye', *Annual of the British School at Athens*, 10: 103–14.

'Londres possède, au British Museum, un ivoire très probablement d'origine grecque . . . et qui nous offre un bel exemple de rachitisme.'

Paul Richer, *L'Art et la Médecine* (Paris, 1902), p. 193

'The hunchback is crouching with his right leg bent under him and his right arm, of which the hand is lost, hanging loosely by his side. His left arm is bent at the elbow and rests on his left knee. The figure is thin and remarkably pigeon-breasted. The collar-bone also is prominent. The head is sunk into the shoulders and leans over towards the left shoulder, which is noticeably lower than the right. The hair is cut very short, the ears are large, the nose aquiline, and great prominence is given to the bone structure above the eyes. In every detail the artist shows an unsparing realism and the most minute observation of an abnormal.'

A. H. S. Yeames, 'An ivory statuette', *Papers of the British School at Rome* 4 (1907), p. 279

'The most important representation of Pott's disease is the beautifully rendered hunchback in the British Museum . . .'

Stevenson, *Pathological Grotesque* (1975), p. 186, cat. no. 145

'We thus have the touchingly realistic figure of a half-nude and weary hunchback slave, apparently found in Italy, now in the British Museum . . .'

R. D. Barnett, *Ancient Ivories in the Middle East* (Jerusalem: Institute of Archaeology, 1982), p. 65

'This skilful ivory carving shows the sad and huddled figure of a slave. He shows signs of dwarfism and a hunch-back, which may be symptoms of Pott's disease. His head drops, and his facial expression is melancholy.

This figure is clearly intended to evoke a sympathetic reaction in the viewer. It is a typical example of the way in which Hellenistic art moved away from idealised representation, and took an interest in the characterization of the individual. The attempt to show personal experience and emotion was applied in both larger-scale sculpture, and in small figures such as this.'

'Ivory figure of a hunchback', British Museum website, 2014

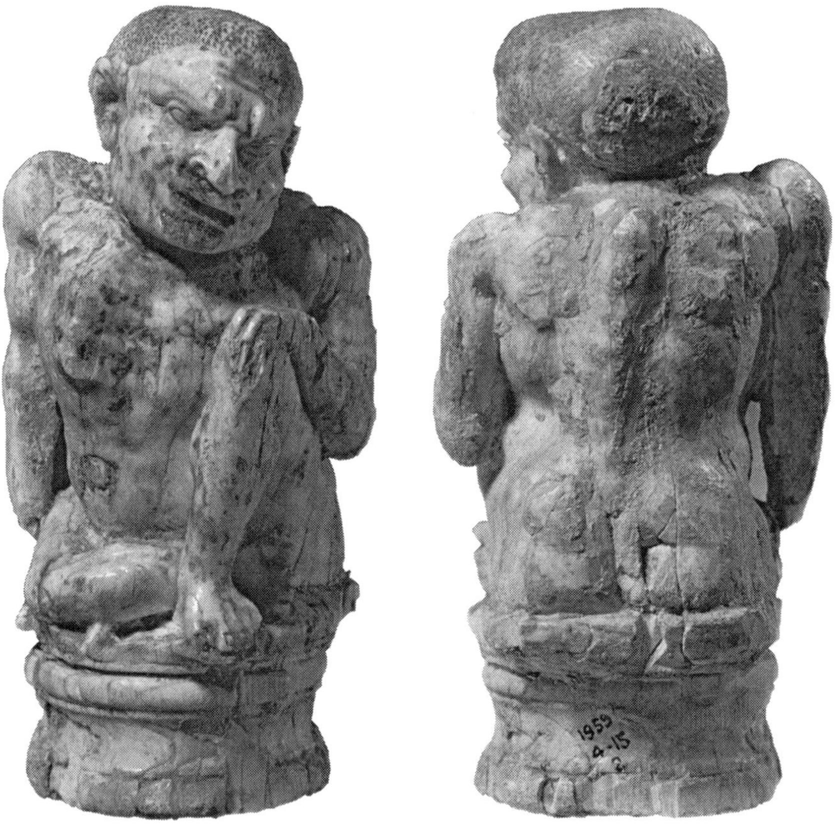

Ivory statuette of a hunchback (cat. no. 40)

London, British Museum. Townley Collection, 1814.7-4.237.
Hellenistic, c. first century BCE.

Introduction

This is a book about *looking* at the Other in Hellenistic and Roman art. More specifically, it is a book about looking at the deformed, and to a lesser extent, the disabled Other using the hunchback as linchpin. But why the hunchback? And why the emphasis on looking?

Corporeal deformity and physical disability has become a topical theme of study, in both the ancient and modern worlds. Aiming to reshape our understanding of culture and identity beyond the 'able' (and by association, the beautiful) body, there have emerged important and ground-breaking works on the history of disability, combined with multiple studies on the representation and reception of deformed and disabled bodies.[1] The figure of the hunchback, however, has, heretofore, received relatively little scholarly attention, resulting in a significant gap in this field of research. This book works towards remedying that.

At the core of this book is a catalogue: a comprehensive collection of hunchback representations, categorized according to formal features, and comprising pieces of different material, date, and diverse provenance, here put together for the first time.[2] The representations in the catalogue form the building blocks for this study; this is where looking becomes critical. To date, scholars have largely *over*looked representations of the hunchback; they have been grouped together and examined in association with other representations of physical deformity (e.g. dwarfs), lacking detailed analysis of the distinct iconography that marks the hunchback as unique. This has resulted in a limited understanding of the varied corpus of Other, and the hunchback in particular. Employing detailed visual analysis of this select group of representations, I focus on the implications of viewing the iconography of the hunchback within the broader context of ancient art and its reception. The focus is not solely on the representations themselves or their meanings: who made them, for whom and why, but the ways in which viewers interact with these representations based on sensory experience, especially sight and touch, so as to understand how viewer engagement contributed to function and meaning. Likewise, a viewer's 'ability' combined with factors such as gender, age, race, ethnicity and social status inevitably affected the reception of these representations; it is these multiple and diverse viewing perspectives that will be examined in the pages that follow. Concomitant with this will be the application of current theory in disability studies to (re)examine the socio-cultural significance of these representations, and, moreover, whenever applicable, attitudes toward the 'real-life' hunchback in Hellenistic and Roman antiquity.

Deformity and disability in contemporary scholarship

This book is the first to examine representations of the hunchback on a rigorous scholarly level; it feeds into a wider, albeit still growing, field addressing the broad topic of corporeal deformity and physical disability in the ancient world. As the subject is still relatively new, it is necessary to trace the work that has been done, and how this present inquiry aims to contribute to the growing body of scholarship.

It was in the early 1990s that the subject of disability in the ancient Greco-Roman world began to arouse the attention of the international academic community, a result, at least in part, of the socio-political climate of the time: the recognition of the disability rights movement that swept over the UK and USA. Recognizing a vast, but relatively un(der)explored corpus of evidence, scholars from diverse backgrounds and disciplines in the arts and sciences have sought to integrate the deformed and disabled body back into our understanding of ancient society and culture, art and representation. This has resulted in a surge in scholarship in recent years.

The first book-length introduction to the topic was Robert Garland's seminal work, *The Eye of the Beholder. Deformity and Disability in the Graeco-Roman World*, which examines how society viewed the deformed and disabled, along with their legal, social and economic status. First published in 1995, a second edition appeared in 2010 with a supplementary bibliography outlining developments in the field. Garland's work spurred a number of subsequent studies: Nicholas Vlahogiannis's *Representations of Disability in the Ancient World* (1998) and his chapters on 'Disabling bodies' in the edited volume by D. Montserrat, *Changing Bodies, Changing Meanings: Studies in the Human Body in Antiquity* (1998) and 'Curing disability' in the edited volume by H. King, *Health in Antiquity* (2005) are especially noteworthy. So too are the contributions of Martha Rose. Her book, *The Staff of Oedipus: Transforming Disability in Ancient Greece* (2003), considers a range of disabilities from the perspective of disability studies, and her entry in the five-volume *Encyclopedia of Disability* (2006), titled 'History of Disability: Ancient West', is the only one of its kind.[3] Most recently, the co-edited Brill volume by C. Laes, C.F. Goodey and M. Rose, *Disabilities in Roman Antiquity: Disparate Bodies A Capite ad Calcem* (2013), representing the first book devoted exclusively to the subject of disability in the ancient Roman world, highlights 'fresh thought, new models of inquiry, and ongoing arguments' (p. 5) within this burgeoning field. So well received was the volume that it is soon to be followed by a Routledge monograph edited by C. Laes on *Disabilities in Antiquity*, scheduled for publication in 2016, which will survey evidence for disability from the Ancient Near East, to Greece and Rome, to the late Antique world and its legacy in comparative, modern world history.

These rather broad surveys have been supplemented by a number of equally important but more narrowly focused efforts, examining specific types of deformities and disabilities in greater detail. The most notable of these include: Dasen's numerous contributions on dwarfs, especially in Egypt and Greece; the many publications by Ajootian on hermaphrodites; Clarke and Versluys' studies on representations of the Aethiops and Egyptian pygmy; Laes' work on deafness; Pestilli's on clubfoot and lameness; Bradley's on obesity; and my own work on blindness.[4] These studies offer a range of methodological approaches to the study of deformity and disability, often combining medical, historical and/or art-historical theory and, of late, disability studies theory, contributing to a more sophisticated understanding of the 'interpretation and representation of the body within the parameters of normality and abnormality' (Vlahogiannis, 2005: 182).

Thus, we have seen in recent years a groundswell of scholarship into deformity and disability in the ancient world, research that has demonstrated the enormous potential of this topic to broaden our understanding of ancient society and culture. Indeed, approaching the ancient world through the lens of deformity and disability adds to a more nuanced understanding of the lives and experiences of the ancients. By examining the figure of the hunchback in Hellenistic and Roman art, this book contributes to a growing scholarly conversation, offering new perspectives on art-historical debates as well as disability studies theory.

The hunchback in contemporary scholarship

This book is intended as a first resource, to fill a critical gap in contemporary scholarship, for representations of the hunchback. Representations of hunchbacks have survived in a variety of media, from small-scale statuettes in terracotta, bronze and ivory, to hanging vases, a vase painting, a wall painting, a mosaic pavement, a bronze mirror and one large-scale marble sculpture. These representations, over fifty in total, have yet to receive formal analysis. Although a select few representations of the hunchback have been studied because of their distinct appearance, the corpus as a whole has never been analysed with any degree of enthusiasm or sophistication.[5] Given the present state of research, this was simply the first work that had to be done. Cataloguing these representations thus provides the foundation for this, and future, study. It is only by *looking* at these representations, individually and as a group, that we can hope to gain a better understanding of the hunchback's complex iconography and its place within the category of Other, and ancient art more generally.

Scholarship on the hunchback in antiquity is limited, and also largely outdated, with the exception of my own work and a very recent publication by Masséglia.[6] To date, the hunchback has been contextualized within the Hellenistic tradition of portraying physical abnormality, the meaning of which is often connected to the grotesque.[7] Numerous interpretations with regards to the function of these grotesques have been put forth, some better received, and indeed convincing, than others. It is worthwhile, therefore, to introduce these interpretations and examine their applicability to the hunchback, which will be done briefly here, and more fully in the chapters that follow.

Since as early as the nineteenth century, scholars have tried to make sense of representations of corporeal deformity and physical disability, attempting to explain and thus legitimize their peculiarity by attributing them specific functions. The earliest of these studies were grounded in the field of medicine, adopting a medical approach to further our understanding of ancient disease and the history of medicine in the West. Many of the scholars studying these representations were either medical practitioners or medical historians who endeavoured to diagnose identifiable pathological conditions represented in these extant ancient works.[8] The clinical accuracy with which some of these pathologies were seemingly represented led some scholars to believe that they functioned as medical teaching aids – though documented evidence of this is lacking, and many of the grotesques are *not* in fact anatomically accurate – while others argued that they were used as prophylactic charms, protecting a healthy individual against the disease they personified or curing them of their condition – though again, evidence to support this is limited.[9]

Representations of the hunchback have thus been contextualized within this medical tradition: documenting spinal pathologies which may have functioned as prophylactic charms. Stevenson, in his 1975 doctoral dissertation, 'The Pathological Grotesque', catalogues 145 representations of osteodystrophic and tubercular pathologies, including rickets, scoliosis, kyphosis and Pott's disease; many of the hunchbacks in our corpus are among those classified by Stevenson. Likewise, the 1998 monograph, *Les Maladies dans l'art Antique*, by co-authors Grmek, a medical doctor and historian, and Gourevitch, a classicist, examines a handful of representations of (our) hunchbacks which are believed to depict specific spinal diseases. These studies have come to dominate our understanding of the hunchback. Indeed, their legacy remains today: some museums still label the hunchback according to the pathology it is believed to possess, for example, the label for the hunchback now in the British Museum (cat. no. **40**) reads: 'A carved ivory figure of a hunchback displaying the symptoms of Pott's disease.'

Although important for understanding the representation of diseases in ancient art, and possibly their diagnosis and treatment, this medical approach fails to address the broader social contexts in which these grotesques were surely displayed and viewed. Following the recognition of the pathological grotesque, archaeologists and art-historians began studying these representations, moving largely, though not completely, away from the medical model, adopting combined historical and/or art-historical approaches, thus attempting to incorporate a wider audience and broader subject matter in their analyses. In 1903, Wace asserted that the majority of grotesques were used as apotropaic charms to ward off the Evil Eye of Envy, since, he argued, ancient evidence suggests that their real-life counterparts were credited with magical powers.[10] In 1913, Richter argued *contra* Wace, identifying grotesque figures with mimic actors, since, she reasoned, they shared with them 'the same bodily deformity, the grimaces, the large phallus, the baldness, the occasional moodiness of expression; in fact a generally ridiculous and coarse appearance'.[11] Still other competing interpretations ensued, including: votives to Asclepius and other divinities, charms to boost sexual potency, and representations of sympotic entertainers or imperial court jesters.[12] However, these interpretations have merely served to downplay and even undermine the cultural importance and aesthetic appeal of these representations. In attempting to explain their oddity, scholars have forgotten that these were objects certainly made for display: representations of hunchbacks decorated both public and private spaces, including bathhouses and villas, throughout the Hellenistic and Roman worlds. A large number of the surviving representations also exhibit extraordinary artistic sophistication and exceptional workmanship. The diverse display contexts and fine quality thus accord these representations a value that scholars have so often failed to recognize: these were objects that had both a practical *and* an aesthetic appeal.

The hunchback in this book

This study takes a rather bold approach, examining key features of the corpus of hunchbacks so as to consider both aesthetic value and practical function. It is organized into four chapters: the first chapter serves as an explanation of the accompanying catalogue and provides a strong visual sense of the range of material under investigation. It examines the different types of hunchback representations, their distinguishing characteristics and the blurring and overlapping between them. The next three chapters examine a series of case studies generated from *looking* at the corpus: Chapter 2 examines the miniature in ancient art, since the vast majority of the representations catalogued are rendered in a miniature format; Chapter 3 examines the phenomenon of hyperphallicism in ancient art, since a large proportion of the hunchbacks catalogued are depicted either with an exaggerated and disproportionately large penis ('macrophallic') or with a prominent erection ('ithyphallic'); and Chapter 4 examines the construction of gender, and corresponding ideas about masculinity and femininity, in ancient art, since all but two of the hunchbacks catalogued are male.

We thus approach the corpus as viewers, considering these representations as individual objects, aiming to reconstruct how they would have been encountered in the ancient world: we examine first their basic size, shape and medium; next, the context(s) in which they were displayed (when known); then we delve deeper into the wider socio-cultural environment in which these representations were viewed.

The vast majority of representations of the hunchback survive as miniature statuettes. Approaching the hunchback, a viewer becomes immediately aware of its small size – small enough, in fact, to fit comfortably into one's hand. Thus invited to pick up the hunchback, the viewer is compelled to touch him and examine him up close for personal delectation. Even out of hand, the small size of the hunchback encourages a viewer to lean in, to look closely so as to inspect the details of his fine representation: the hump of the hunchback becomes the point of focus, with its smooth or ridged surface – another tactile invitation, tempting a viewer to rub the hunchback's hump. Continuing the inspection, a viewer is met with the face and body of a man, one with a disproportionately large (and sometimes erect) penis. Other features, too, draw the viewer's attention: a body often contorted in awkward positions, both standing and seated, and a pitiful expression revealing a sullen mood or one of pain and suffering. Sometimes the hunchback has large, penetrating eyes and gazes directly at the viewer, imploring him/her to stop and stare; other times the hunchback looks down or away, cowering from the viewer's gaze. All of these features, and more, demand that the viewer *engage* with the hunchback, to both look *and* touch, and in so doing, force the viewer to question the meaning ascribed to the body of the hunchback. This, in turn, prompts the viewer to reflect upon the meaning of his/her own (ab/normal) body, thus potentially blurring the boundaries between Self and Other.

Viewer engagement is an equally important component of the few representations in the corpus that survive in other media, that is, not as miniature statuettes. The wall painting and mosaic pavement (cat. nos **16** and **17**, respectively) are intended to be looked at, but they too demand that a viewer lean in or crouch down to get the best view of the hunchback. In both representations the gaze of the hunchback directs that of the viewer, drawing him/her into the scene, creating a narrative by making the viewer imagine what has already happened and/or what will happen next. But in as much as these representations encourage the viewer to engage, they also, by virtue of their two-dimensionality, ensure that the viewer remains at a distance, thus maintaining the role of an outsider looking in and affirming the difference between Self and Other. The bronze vase and bronze mirror (cat. nos **20** and **41**, respectively), on the other hand, play out the ways in which multiple viewers could engage simultaneously with a single viewed object. Not only meant to be looked at, these were objects that, as part of their practical function, were intended to be hand-held and used. Physically holding the vase in one's hand to empty its contents allowed not only the primary be-holder to admire its decorative scenes, but also other viewers as well; likewise, holding the mirror in one's hand, so that the primary viewer could admire his/her reflection, allowed other viewers to observe the hunchback on the reverse. Like the hunchback in miniature, the combination of optic and haptic encounter created a rich and varied multi-sensory viewing experience. Furthermore, the contexts of all of these representations, namely how and where they were displayed, not only force a viewer to question their function, but also, to consider the place of the hunchback in contemporary society.

Thus, the chapters that follow assess the importance of the hunchback in Hellenistic and Roman art, and, in so doing, address broader issues in ancient representation, such as miniaturization and hyperphallicism, which, much like the hunchback, have been marginalized or inadequately studied in contemporary scholarship. By challenging traditional hierarchies that lie at the very heart of ancient representation, this study provides a way of re-thinking and re-reading images of the Other in Hellenistic and Roman art, using the hunchback as linchpin.

A note to readers: the catalogue of hunchbacks and accompanying plates follow immediately after the conclusion but should not be left until the end for perusal. Readers are invited to *look* for themselves, now, and while reading each of the chapters that follow, and in their looking will hopefully find additional layers of meaning in the representation of the hunchback.

1

What's in a Hump? Representing the Hunchback

The accompanying catalogue collects fifty-five representations of hunchbacks from the Hellenistic and Roman worlds; these representations vary in material, size, date, and provenance, but are connected in the visual record by one distinct iconographic feature: a hump protruding from each figure's back. This hump can vary in size and shape: it can be a smooth, compact, rounded hump (e.g. cat. nos **2**, **4**, **8**, **9**, **10**, **16–19** and **44**) or it can be a ridged hump, with the thoracic vertebrae clearly articulated and looking like a dorsal 'fin' (e.g. cat. nos **11–15**, **33–7**, **40**, **41** and **48**), or it can be an angular hump, in that it protrudes outward *and* upward (e.g. cat. nos **3**, **20**, **22–7**, **30**, **45–7** and **50**). In two-dimensional representation, the hump of the hunchback is always round; in three-dimensional representation, however, artists experimented with a wider variety of shapes, thus creating a different look, and indeed feel, for each hump. Regardless of medium (statuette, mosaic pavement or vase painting), the hunchback always possesses marked spinal curvature which causes a protuberance from the back, whether mild or significant, thus making his identity immediately recognizable.

Despite this rather obvious iconographic feature, numerous representations have, in the past, been misidentified as hunchbacks. Indeed, a number of representations that other scholars have labelled as hunchbacks have been excluded from this catalogue altogether. For example, Ruffer, Bieber and Fowler have identified a representation of a dancing dwarf in the Metropolitan Museum of Art in New York as a hunchback (Figure 1).[1] Upon closer inspection, however, and when viewed in comparison with some of the far more obvious examples of hunchbacks in our corpus, it is clear that this dwarf does not have a visible hump or marked spinal curvature. Rather, what is represented is

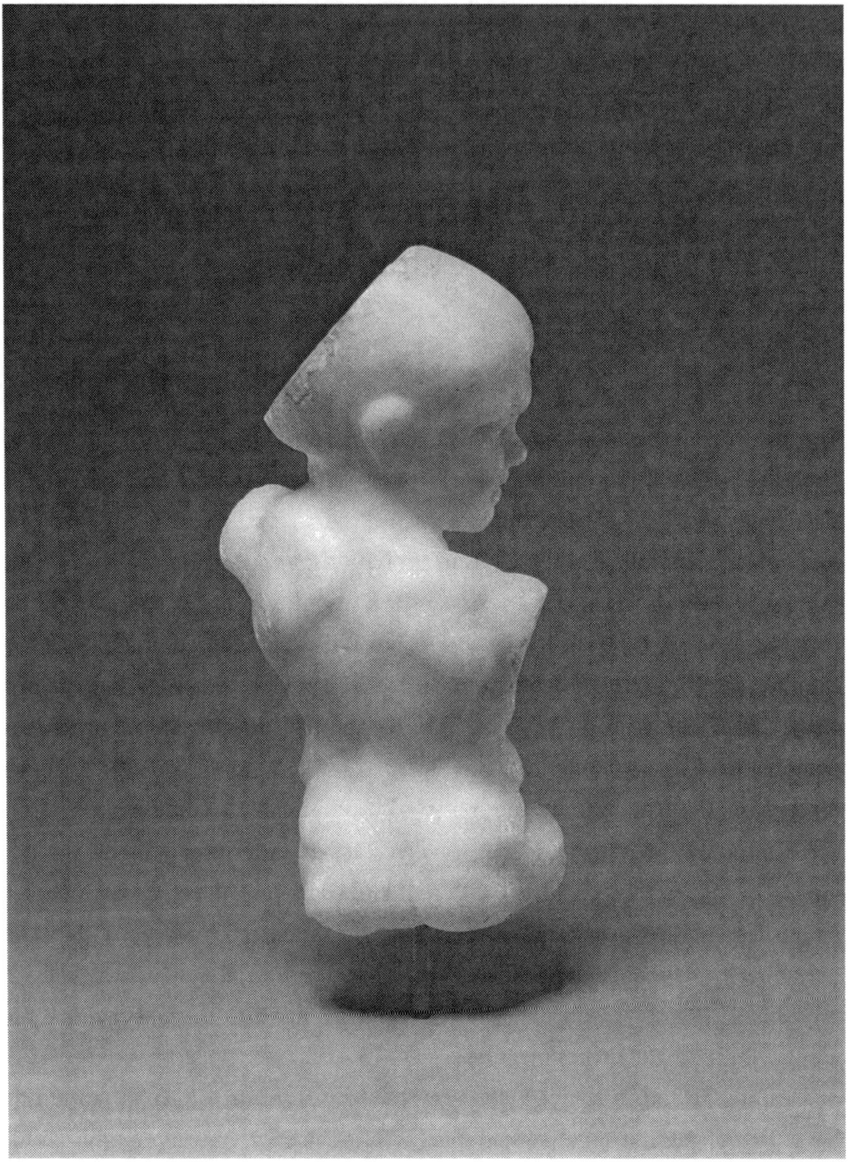

Figure 1 Marble statuette of a dancing dwarf, c. third to first century BCE. Metropolitan Museum of Art, New York, 26.7.1403.

defined dorsal musculature, revealing the movements of a body in motion, highlighting the torsional pose of this dancing dwarf. Part of the error in identification seems to be the blurring in iconography between the dwarf and the hunchback (more on this below), and a poor understanding of each of these different types. Likewise, misidentification can occur, since, as we shall soon see, looking can, at times, prove difficult. Therefore, before moving directly to the classification of the hunchback, it is necessary to briefly outline the challenges of the analysis that follows.

The catalogue and its challenges

In analysing the catalogue of hunchbacks, a number of methodological difficulties were encountered which have inevitably influenced this study. Perhaps the most considerable of these is the lack of provenance for the majority of hunchback representations: this is due to the fact that they were principally discovered during uncontrolled excavations and have often changed hands several times between excavators, collectors and museums. Often, even when a general provenance is known, no details as to the exact location of the find-spot are provided. Out of the fifty-five representations catalogued, twenty-nine have a general provenance recorded.[2] Of these twenty-nine, only seven have a secure archaeological context; however, the exact location within these areas is often unclear.[3] For example, although the hunchback now in the Villa Albani-Torlonia (cat. no. **32**), the sole surviving large-scale sculpture in the corpus, was discovered in the Baths of Caracalla in Rome, where and how it would have been displayed within the Baths remains uncertain, since archaeological reports state only that it was found among a hoard of other sculptures in a building addition to the Baths. Likewise, the wall painting discovered in Pompeii (cat. no. **16**) has no details as to its find-spot recorded (was it a villa, a brothel or a public bath?) and the painting no longer survives.[4] The only representation for which the context is accurately documented is the mosaic pavement decorating the north vestibule leading to a portico and garden at a Roman villa in Jekmejeh, near Antioch (cat. no. **17**).

Notwithstanding the unknown provenance of the majority of hunchback representations, many of the terracotta statuettes have been attributed to the workshops of Alexandria in Egypt and Smyrna in Asia Minor, since it is here that representations of grotesques have survived in large numbers. The attribution of these representations to such locations is, however, tenuous; especially problematic are those attributed to Smyrna. Virtually all of the grotesques recovered from Smyrna were found during illicit excavations and survive in fragments; often heads of figurines or headless torsos and separate limbs. The origin of these fragments is enigmatic: initially believed to have originated from a cemetery, then later from the ruins of houses, the most recent suggestion is that they may have been part of a large votive deposit (Higgins 1967: 110). Without context, these terracottas are bound by their style and technique, distinct to Smyrna with generally orange- or pale orange-coloured clay with a fine shiny surface and a grey core, and occasionally decorated with a yellow or green lead glaze. A number of the terracotta hunchbacks in the corpus which have been attributed to Smyrna do not correspond with these stylistic or technical qualities: the fabric and heavy white slip of two statuettes (cat. nos **30** and **52**) are anomalous among the corpus of terracottas from the site, but are rather characteristic of terracottas from Boeotia. Of the remaining representations, only one (cat. no. **55**) appears in the distinct orange clay typical of Smyrnaean terracottas.

Due to the fact that the majority of hunchback representations lack a secure provenance, dating them is also challenging. Even those with a secure archaeological context can be problematic. For example, as mentioned above, the hunchback now in the Villa Albani-Torlonia (cat. no. **32**) was discovered in the Baths of Caracalla in Rome. Although dated to the second century CE on the basis of its hairstyle and drilling technique, whether it is a creation of its time or a copy of some now lost Greek original has been the cause of significant debate. The sculpture has been identified as a Roman copy of a Greek original representing the famous Greek fabulist Aesop, based primarily on literary sources that report that a statue of the fabulist existed in Athens in the fifth century BCE. However, none of these sources describe the statue, and no inscription survives to positively identify it, thus it is impossible to determine whether that rumoured sculpture of Aesop was similar in appearance to the bust in the Villa Albani-Torlonia.[5]

The increased interest of Hellenistic artists in the grotesque body starting in the third century BCE suggests a general *terminus post quem* for the majority of hunchback representations; however, it is often difficult to determine whether these representations are Hellenistic originals or Roman 'copies'. Evidence from Delos and Pompeii suggests that the production and popularity of grotesques flourished between the first century BCE and the first century

CE, although individual pieces are often given broad date ranges spanning from the third century BCE to the second century CE, and many of those attributed a Hellenistic date could equally be Roman. For example, the miniature bronze hunchback now in the Museum für Kunst und Gewerbe in Hamburg (cat. no. **33**), which makes several appearances in the chapters that follow, has been dated to the third century BCE on the tacit assumption that its high quality indicates an early, and thus Hellenistic, date. It could, however, based on its shared iconography with the hunchback now in the Antikensammlung in Berlin (cat. no. **34**), be dated to the Roman period. It is therefore almost impossible to fix a secure chronology for the iconographic development of the hunchback. Consequently, this study makes no attempt at periodization, which may, to the traditional archaeologist and art historian, seem disagreeable; this has implications for how these images were viewed, but efforts have been made to contextualize these representations within the wider spectrum of Hellenistic and Roman art.

The lack of provenance and imprecise dates for hunchback representations is but one problem encountered in their study. A number of additional problems emerged while examining details of the figures themselves, particularly with regards to their current state of preservation. The present visual image of the hunchback is markedly different from what these figures would have looked like – and therefore how they would have been viewed and received – in antiquity.

The surviving corpus of hunchback representations is primarily confined to a miniature format. As such, issues concerning fragmentation and the effects of restoration are significantly less, though not eliminated. Fifteen out of the fifty-five representations of hunchbacks suffer minor fragmentation, while eight survive as a bust or torso. Of these, often the arms, legs or hands are missing, likely because, as extremities, these were most susceptible to damage during handling, transportation, burial or recovery. With regards to restoration, the large-scale marble sculpture of the hunchback now in the Villa Albani-Torlonia (cat. no. **32**) is the only representation in the corpus that has been significantly restored: the nose, right shoulder and back of the head are all restorations and the leg stumps, like the semi-erect penis which is now covered by a fig leaf, were smoothly worked off and smeared with plaster. On the whole, the corpus of hunchbacks is fairly well preserved, especially compared to other corpuses of ancient sculpture where fragmentation and restoration have had a more direct and visible effect.

Despite the fact that relatively few representations in the corpus are fragmented or restored, representations of hunchbacks nonetheless reveal the effects of having survived their journey from antiquity. The dull, brownish surface and worn details of the terracotta statuettes (now often deemed 'crude' art because of their appearance) were often brightly painted in antiquity, as evidenced by traces of paint on cat. nos **10**, **30** and **52**. Likewise, the dark patina of the bronze statuettes would have once gleamed gold, appearing even more elaborate when coupled with silver inlay, as evidenced on cat. nos **8**, **9**, **12** and **33**. Finally, the ivory used for the hunchback now in the British Museum (cat. no. **40**), presently dulled and darkened, would have originally appeared luminously white, perhaps even reminding an ancient viewer of some of the most famous ivory works of antiquity, known through both art and literature.

Analysis of the current state of these representations was also compromised on account of the poor quality of available photographs. The majority of published photographs of the hunchback were taken early in the nineteenth century and appear in black and white, which blurs details and obscures features. More problematic is the fact that these photographs often show limited viewpoints; many do not show the back of the figure, the hunchback's hump, the key identifier of the hunchback. As such, new photographs were requested and, in some cases, but unfortunately not all, obtained and have been included here. Viewing these objects in their respective museums, whenever possible and if accessible to the public, was the primary tool of analysis for this study. Any errors in identification, though always checked against other sources, are, of course, my own.

The problems encountered in examining the corpus of hunchback representations does not undermine its value for study; rather, it demonstrates that a thorough examination has been long overdue. As a figure that has received so little scholarly attention, the hunchback provides a new and rich source for investigation into deformity and disability in antiquity. Furthermore, looking at this corpus anew will reveal much about the production and consumption of ancient art in the Hellenistic and Roman worlds. So now, to the catalogue.

The structure of the catalogue

The catalogue is divided into three main sections. The first two are based on pose, for the reason that all representations of hunchbacks are depicted either standing or sitting. These two sections are further sub-divided based on (1) clothing, where the hunchback is depicted either nude, semi-nude with only a loincloth, or draped by a simple tunic; and (2) actions, where the hunchback appears involved in some kind of performance; either dancing, playing an instrument or ritual sacrificing. The third section consists of fragments of hunchbacks, in the form of busts and/or torsos. Due to the fragmented condition of these representations it is impossible to reconstruct their pose with confidence; they could not, therefore, be incorporated into the preceding two sections. In all categories, there are clear iconographic similarities that connect these representations and extend beyond the hunchback's main identifying feature, the hump.

Perhaps the most glaring aspect of the corpus of hunchbacks is related to their gender: all but two representations of the hunchback are male; we shall explore some of the causes and consequences of this gendered representation in Chapter 4. The male hunchback is almost always depicted with generic, sometimes grotesque, facial features and an emotive expression. In a small group of examples (cat. nos **9**, **17**, **32**, **48**, **49** and **52**), these generic features are replaced by a portrait-style head, which may indicate an attempt to portray a particular individual, rather than a type. With regards to body type, the hunchback is typically represented with elongated limbs and an emaciated body, a large, bald head, or a top/side-knot of hair, and a large or erect phallus.[6] Occasionally, the elongated character of the hunchback's body is replaced by dwarfed limbs and a shortened trunk. With regards to clothing, the hunchback is most often depicted either nude or semi-nude with only a loincloth around his waist; however, in two examples, the hunchbacks now in the Metropolitan Museum of Art in New York (cat. no. **8**) and the Walters Art Gallery in Baltimore (cat. no. **9**), the hunchback wears a costume consisting of a tunic, through which the hump remains clearly visible. On occasion, the hunchback also wears a (pointed) cap, a brimmed hat, or what appears to be a wreath of leaves.

In terms of pose, representations of hunchbacks form two distinct compositional groups where the position of viewer and figure alike appear to have been carefully manipulated: the standing or stooping hunchback and the seated or crouching hunchback. Representations of hunchbacks standing or stooping constitute the largest group of figures in the assemblage; thirty are depicted in this manner compared to the fifteen depicted seated or crouching. In both groups, the pose serves to highlight as starkly as possible (whether in two or three dimensions) the hunchback's most outstanding physical attribute: the hump. In all representations, the hunchback's identity is immediately recognizable because the hump is the most prominent physical feature on display.

Within the standing group twelve representations depict the hunchback carrying an object. The majority of these representations (seven out of twelve) depict the hunchback carrying a cockerel and a *lagynos*, or wine-jug. The hunchback carries the cockerel in his right arm and, with head angled, stares at the cockerel demurely. In four examples (cat. nos **22**, **23**, **25** and **26**), the cockerel appears to be pecking at the hunchback's face but fails to provoke a reaction. In his hanging left hand the hunchback carries a *lagynos*. Two of these representations (cat. nos **22** and **23**) show the hunchback sporting a distinct double beard, split in the middle, which occasionally appears in representations of mimic actors. This group of representations have been interpreted as votives to the god Asclepius, on the basis that the hunchback carries a sacrificial animal and libation; problematically, however, none of these representations have been found in votive contexts.[7]

The object held by the hunchback in the five remaining representations is more obscure. In these representations the object(s) cannot be positively identified, although we might assume it to be a cockerel and/or a vase, based on the examples just discussed, or a bag, based on representations of the seated hunchback who, on occasion, carries a bag over his shoulder (see below). In only one representation, the hunchback now in the Museum of Fine Arts in Boston (cat. no. **30**), is the object recognizable. Here, the hunchback carries a bunch of grapes at groin level. The provenance of this figure is reportedly Smyrna; however, a comparable figurine of a dwarf eating grapes also now in the Museum of Fine Arts in Boston originates from Anthedon in Boeotia (Figure 2). Both figures are decorated with a heavy white slip and the grapes they carry are hand-modelled. These figures recall images of the god Priapus who sometimes appears carrying fruit, stressing his association with fertility

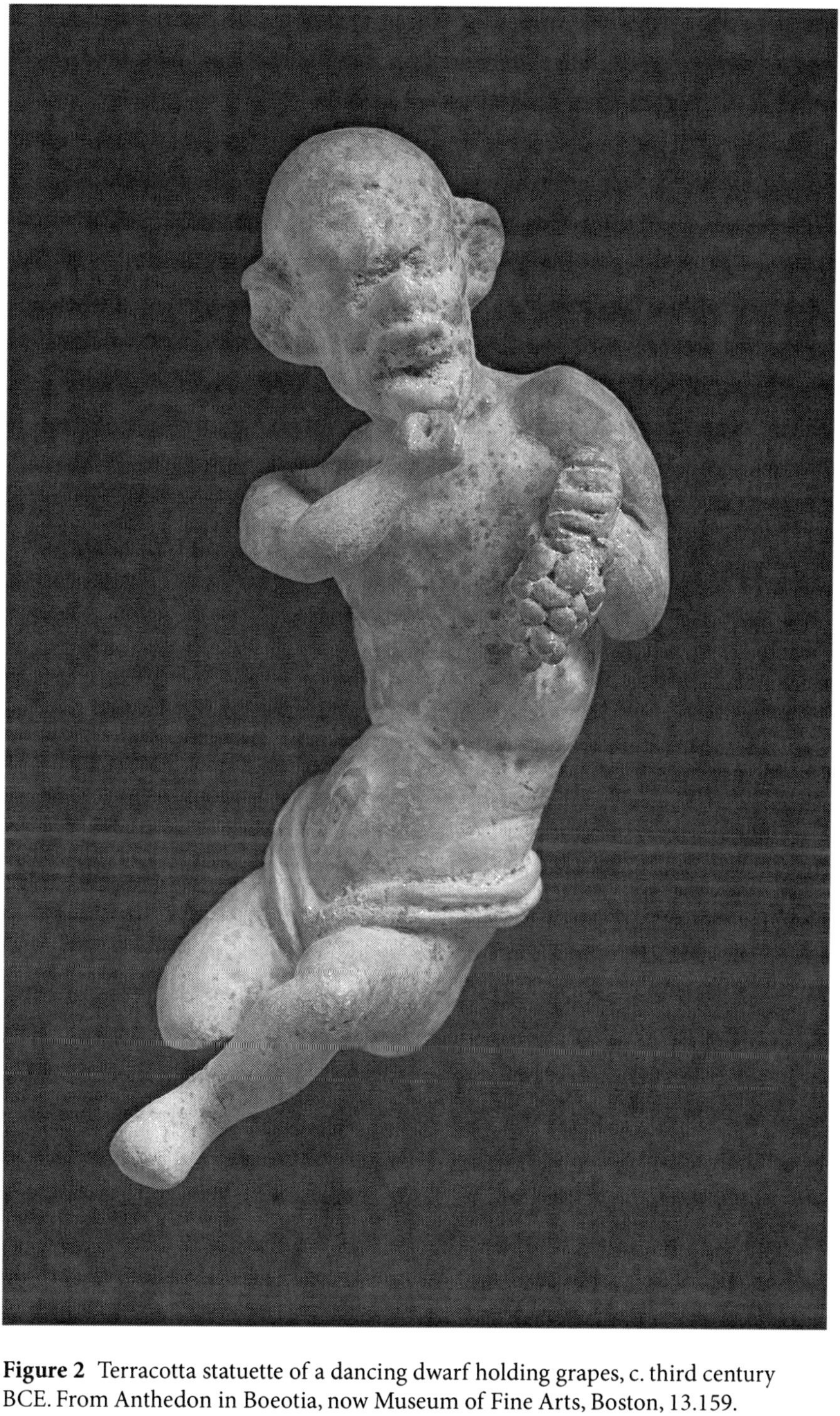

Figure 2 Terracotta statuette of a dancing dwarf holding grapes, c. third century BCE. From Anthedon in Boeotia, now Museum of Fine Arts, Boston, 13.159.

and fecundity. The extent this association can be applied to the hunchback, however, is uncertain, since there are only two such figures (see below for the other, seated, figure, cat. no. **46**) depicted carrying fruit.

Representations of hunchbacks dancing are restricted to a small group consisting of five statuettes, one wall painting and one mosaic pavement. Of these, two examples (cat. nos **12** and **17**) are characterized by their torsional pose; the hunchback steps forward on his right foot with head turned back, looking over his right shoulder. Two of these dancing figures (cat. nos **16** and **17**) also carry rhythm sticks.[8] These sticks appear frequently in ancient representations of dancing figures; held one in each hand, they were used chiefly as an idiophone (an instrument that creates sound from the vibration of the instrument as a whole) to mark rhythm and for emphasizing the poses in the dance; in representations of the hunchback, these sticks may also have served an added talismanic function by making noise and thus frightening the forces of evil.

Another small group of representations, consisting of two statuettes and one vase painting, depict the hunchback playing an instrument. The two statuettes (cat. nos **18** and **19**) may have once played the double-flute or perhaps held rhythm sticks. The hunchback depicted on a bronze vase (cat. no. **20**) is dressed in a loincloth and pointed cap and plays the double-flute. This hunchback is accompanied by three other dwarf figures, all similarly dressed and performing various tasks at what appears to be a feast. The scene suggests that the hunchback is part of an entertaining troupe. In addition to this group, one representation categorized as carrying a cockerel (cat. no. **24**) may also have been depicted playing the castanet, though this object cannot be identified with certainty because of its partial preservation.

In the second compositional group of seated or crouching hunchbacks, the hunchback is often depicted seated on a rock in a near-foetal position.[9] With head tilted downward and wearing an emotive expression, these hunchbacks are either grimacing in pain and suffering or are timid and fearful. By reducing himself to a near-foetal position, the hunchback appears to cower from the viewer, withdrawing himself from the spectator's gaze. This pose, with slight variations, was popularly used by Hellenistic artists in the representation of slaves and may serve to highlight the hunchback's social inferiority as well as sub-human status; this will be explored further in Chapter 4.

Within the seated or crouching group, the hunchback also appears riding an animal, identified as a donkey or goat, as in cat. nos **46** and **47**. On both figures, the humps are angular and pointed and the heads are richly modelled with full brows, noses and mouths. Catalogue no. **46** also carries fruit, possibly grapes similar to cat. no. **30**. Uhlenbrock has suggested that these two figures, along with cat. no. **29**, may have been products of the same unknown centre and formed a group, because of their conceptual and stylistic similarities; however, as the provenance and dates of all three statuettes are unknown, such an assertion must remain purely speculative (Uhlenbrock 1990: 162). Other seated hunchbacks are also represented carrying an object, but these are far fewer in number than in representations of the standing and stooping hunchback: in addition to cat. no. **46** which carries fruit, cat. no. **37** holds a string or leather thong to infibulate his large penis, cat. no. **41** holds a bird in the palm of his hand, cat. no. **44** carries a bag over his shoulder, and cat. no. **45** carries a *kantharos*, a drinking cup, usually for wine.

In addition to the standing and seated hunchbacks listed above, two hunchbacks in the corpus appear in the form of miniature hanging vases (cat. nos **48** and **49**). Both figures are represented with portrait-style faces and one figure (cat. no. **48**) wears a wreath atop his head.[10] These hanging hunchbacks are part of a relatively small group of similar miniature bronzes that survive predominantly from Egypt; these have been variously interpreted as balsam containers which may have stored oil or perfumes for use at baths, or as sympotic decorations, or as funerary votives (Perdrizet 1911: 59–60, no. 96). We shall examine these interpretations in further detail in Chapter 2.

In terms of size and material, the majority of hunchback representations (fifty out of fifty-five) are represented in three dimension, that is to say in the form of statues, restricted to a miniature format, ranging from 5.1 centimetres to 19.0 centimetres in height, and survive chiefly in bronze and terracotta. Their miniature size suggests an intimate relationship with the viewer; the viewer can engage in 'active' viewing, handling the statuette, feeling its contours, and moving it around in order to examine it from any angle. Six of these miniatures (cat. nos **5**, **15**, **38**, **45**, **48** and **49**) are equipped with suspension holes or loops which indicate that they were meant to be hung either from the body or from a building. The remaining two-dimensional representations, the wall painting, mosaic pavement, vase painting and bronze mirror, can all be associated with a private (domestic) context, which affirms a personal, intimate viewing environment for these images. Only one large-scale sculpture of a hunchback survives, the marble hunchback now in the Villa Albani-Torlonia in Rome (cat. no. **32**). This representation is also important because it has the most detailed portrait head and a secure archaeological context: it was found in the Baths of Caracalla in Rome. As the only representation in the corpus that is firmly associated with a public display space, its viewing context is obviously different from the miniature hunchback; we will explore this in more detail in Chapter 2.

The surviving visual record reveals that there existed a wide and varied repertoire for the possible stylistic representation of the hunchback. The prototype for these representations – whether it was a large-scale sculpture or a statuette – and the form that this took, however, remains uncertain. The literary and epigraphic evidence also reveals little about the production or display of these images. It is therefore imperative that *looking* at the corpus of hunchbacks is central to its analysis. Indeed, looking at the corpus reveals a number of links between the hunchback, the Other and even the body beautiful. It is thus useful to briefly examine some of these connections to further nuance our understanding of the representation of the hunchback.

The hunchback and the Other

A look at the catalogue reveals a number of iconographic and stylistic similarities between the hunchback and other representations of the Other. Examples within this broad category of Other range from some of the more pretty or alluring hermaphrodites, to the more mundane, everyday emaciated men and obese women, to the physically deformed dwarf, to the foreign black African. The blurring between these images and intentional elision in iconography is important in thinking about how these images work as a group, and can be used to help inform the meaning of the hunchback. Here follows a general overview of the hunchback's connection(s) to the Other; direct comparisons using specific examples will be deployed in subsequent chapters.

Perhaps the most recognizable feature of the corpus is that representations of hunchbacks can appear dwarfed in corporeal proportion or possess certain black African features. Out of the fifty-five representations of hunchbacks catalogued nine (cat. nos **1**, **3**, **4**, **7**, **30**, **33–5** and **40**) are represented with African features, such as black skin (indicated by a shiny black patina), thick lips and flat noses with broad nostrils; nine (cat. nos **3**, **7**, **16**, **17**, **20**, **30**, **32**, **45** and **55**) are represented as hunchbacked dwarfs, characterized by their long trunks, short limbs and disproportionately large heads; and four (cat. nos **3**, **7**, **16** and **30**) are represented as dwarfed, African hunchbacks.[11] Clearly the blurring in iconography is intentional.

One iconographic feature in particular seems to link representations of the hunchback, black African and dwarf: their hyperphallicism. All three of these types are commonly depicted with exaggeratedly large or erect penises. In the corpus of hunchbacks, thirty figures are represented in this manner. Garmaise catalogues fifty dwarfs in statuette form similarly represented, and it is certain that this number would be higher if it were to include the numerous representations of dwarfs depicted on vase paintings and wall paintings (Garmaise, *Dwarfs*, 128–9). Although no similar calculation has been made with regard to the black African, one distinct group of representations is invariably represented in this way; those ithyphallic swimmers and macrophallic bath attendants appearing on mosaic pavements in Pompeian baths and Roman baths of North Africa, popular during the imperial period (Clarke, esp. 1996). The frequency with which these figures are represented as hyperphallic suggests that this attribute is a critical iconographic pointer in accessing the function and meaning of these images; the hyperphallic nature of the hunchback will thus be the focus of Chapter 3.

Not only do representations of the hunchback, black African and dwarf share a number of similar corporeal features, but there is also extensive overlap in their poses, which themselves draw upon representations of the body beautiful. In Classical Greece, the body beautiful was always portrayed in an ideal, youthful state, without wrinkles, blemishes or imperfections, and came to stand as the canon against which all art was later measured.[12] It is surely significant that many Hellenistic and Roman representations of the Other are directly based upon, and often parody, specific sculptural types of the body beautiful, such as the dancing figures and those in the pose of a Spinario, suggesting that their very iconography demanded a viewer make explicit associations and connections.

The Other and the body beautiful

A look at the catalogue also reveals a number of iconographic and stylistic similarities between the hunchback and representations of the body beautiful. Seven representations in the corpus depict the hunchback dancing. Of these, two examples (cat. nos **12** and **17**) are characterized by their torsional pose; the hunchback steps forward on his right foot with head turned back, looking over his right shoulder. This pose is also common among representations of dancing dwarfs (Figure 3), which have traditionally been interpreted as caricatures of the many elegant dancing female figures of Greek art and/or religious dancers employed at festivals and banquets, specifically in honour of Dionysus.[13]

Representations of dancing figures on vase paintings and in sculptural form abound from the ancient world.[14] Although the poses of such dancing figures vary considerably, the turning of the figure's head, usually looking over its shoulder, is one of the most repeated, and thus distinguishing, features. It is a particularly important feature in representations of *Aphrodite Kallipygos*, or 'Beautiful-Bottom'.[15] In these representations the goddess of sex and sexual love flaunts her beauty and is presented as an object of erotic display. The goddess is depicted semi-exposed; although she wears a long garment to conceal her body, she lifts it up and away from herself to reveal her bared buttocks, a movement which causes her right shoulder strap to fall, exposing part of her right breast, thus further heightening her sexual attraction. Looking back over her right shoulder and admiring her own bottom, she leads the viewer's gaze there too, and thus invites him/her to admire it also.

The dancing hunchback seems to employ a similar pose to that of Aphrodite, drawing attention to his outstanding physical feature, the prominent hump on his back. Though the hunchback does not flaunt his body in the same way as the goddess Aphrodite, his deformity is nevertheless put on display. By turning to look at his hump, the viewer's gaze and attention are also brought there. What implication(s) would such an association have had upon an ancient viewer? Might the hump of a hunchback also prompt an erotic response or arouse desire in a viewer? A passage in Pliny (*NH* 34. 6. 12), which will be discussed in detail in Chapter 3, certainly suggests this possibility and perhaps taps into a common (though subversive) theme of deformity having an erotic appeal.[16]

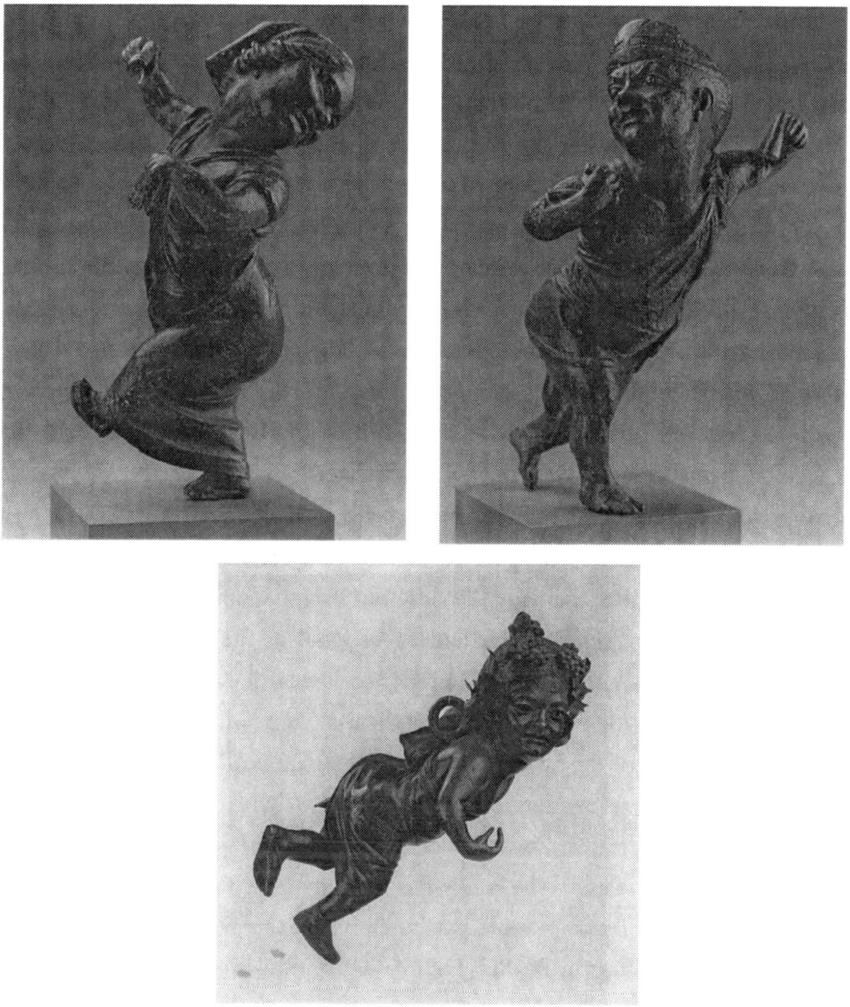

Figure 3 Bronze statuettes of dancing dwarfs, c. mid-second century BCE. From the Mahdia shipwreck, now Bardo National Museum, Tunis, F213, F214, F215.

More than this (potentially) erotic association, there is another important aspect in the repeated poses of the aforementioned figures: these two types represent extreme opposites in appearance, the goddess of beauty and the deformed Other, and thus served to normalize the viewer by asking him/her where he/she would fit on a sliding scale of divine and debased. Both goddess and Other are presented as the antitheses of normality; part of their appeal surely arises from the viewer's recognition of the ease with which they could slide unsteadily into one another.

In addition to the dancing figures, two representations in the corpus, the hunchback now in the Wadsworth Atheneum in Connecticut (cat. no. **35**) and the hunchback now in the Louvre in Paris (cat. no. **36**), appear in the pose of a Spinario, or thorn-puller. The hunchback in the Wadsworth Atheneum (cat. no. **35**) is seated on a rock, hunched over with his right leg crossed over the left, examining his foot. He is nude except for a pointed cap, which is similar to the cap worn by the hunchback playing the double-flute depicted on the bronze vase (cat. no. **20**). He has thin, elongated limbs and possesses African features, including a snub nose. The hunchback in the Louvre (cat. no. **36**) is also seated, though his original (rocky) base is now missing. He too is hunched over but with his left leg crossed over the right. Although attempting to extract the thorn from his left foot, he appears to gaze elsewhere, to his right. He is nude and extremely emaciated, but with remarkably well-defined musculature.

Different versions of the Spinario have survived from antiquity, in bronze, marble and terracotta, each slightly different in appearance but all ostensibly derived from an early Greek Hellenistic original of the third century BCE. A bronze version in the Palazzo dei Conservatori in Rome, representing a nude, idealized youth with an early classical-style head, is the most famous surviving example of the Spinario.[17] A marble figure in the British Museum in London, also nude, is rendered more realistically than the bronze figure, but still has classical features, and appears to have functioned as a fountain, indicated by two holes in the rocky base and evident wearing from water.[18] Differing significantly from these two versions is a terracotta Spinario now in the Antikensammlung in Berlin (Figure 4).[19] Found in a villa at Priene and dated between the second and first century BCE, the figure is depicted wearing a peasant cap and tattered tunic fastened on his left shoulder. He has ugly, caricatured features, possesses black African characteristics, including thick lips and a flat nose with broad nostrils, and has a large phallus. As an uglier and later version, it is important to note that this Spinario is represented in miniature, measuring 16.8 centimetres in height. His physical features and size place him iconographically and stylistically closer to the hunchback in our corpus, and both are visually at odds with the other versions. These two latter figures belong to the realm of grotesques and exist in small scale, sharply contrasting the idealism of the other near life-size Spinario figures.

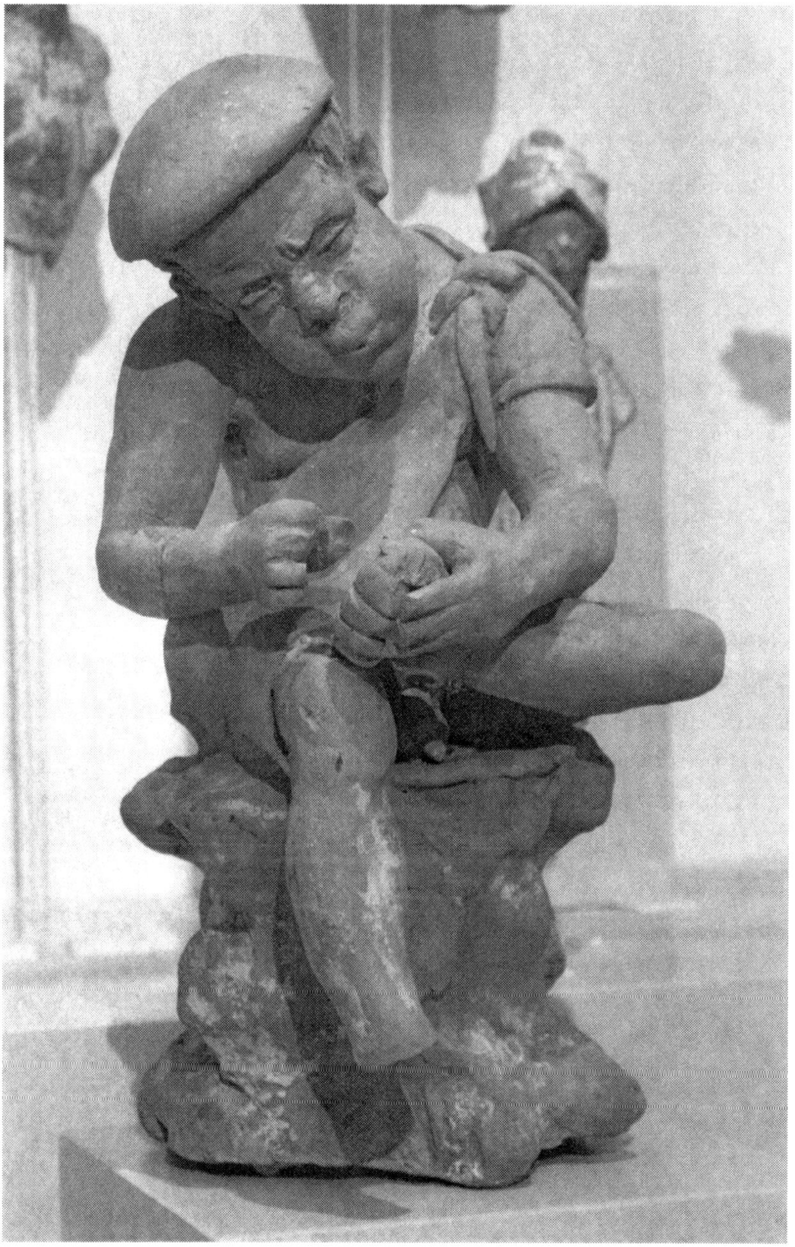

Figure 4 Terracotta statuette of a Spinario, c. second to first century BCE. From Priene, House 33 East, now Antikensammlung Staatliche Museum, Berlin, TC 8626.

What are the implications of representing such diverse types in the same pose? What associations would an ancient viewer have made? The thorn-in-foot motif was popular for both single figures and group compositions (e.g. Pan and satyrs) in the Hellenistic period and has been variously interpreted.[20] The Priene statuette too has received much attention, interpreted both as 'a parody of the dignified original' and 'a sympathetic study of a racial type'.[21] As Masséglia has recently argued, these rustic peasants are otherized not just by their physical ugliness, but by the fact that they are uncivilized in their behaviour when compared to non-rustics performing the same activity.[22] Thus, similar to the dancing figures above, the variance between the idealized and grotesque Spinario suggests a sliding scale between beautiful and ugly, ideal and non-ideal, civilized and uncivilized, demanding that a viewer question his/her own status and normality against these different (but the same) types.

By outlining some of the blurring and overlapping in iconography between representations of the hunchback, the Other and the body beautiful, it has become clear that the neat categories modern scholars affix to such diverse images were by no means as clearly delineated in antiquity. Indeed, artists seem to have relished blurring the boundaries between these different types to stress both difference *and* similarity. The chapters that follow will demonstrate in further detail, and through a variety of additional examples, the extent of this blurring and how this inevitably impacted a viewer's response to the hunchback.

2

Multum in Parvo: The Hunchback in Miniature

The vast majority of representations of the hunchback survive as miniature statuettes: of the fifty-five representations catalogued, fifty are rendered in miniature, ranging in height from 5.1 centimetres to 19.0 centimetres.[1] These miniatures do not derive from a large-scale original, nor is there a single, identifiable prototype for their production; indeed, only one large-scale sculpture of a hunchback survives, the hunchback now in the Villa Albani-Torlonia (cat. no. **32**). This is by no means unusual; looking beyond the hunchback, representations of the Other, especially the deformed and disabled Other (e.g. the dwarf), also survive chiefly as miniature statuettes. Why did artists choose to confine the Other to a miniature scale and how did these miniatures appeal to consumers?

This chapter will explore the sculptural production and reception of the miniature in ancient art by deploying detailed analysis of the hunchback in miniature. We begin with an evaluation of the aesthetic appeal of these objects as display pieces, examining the processes involved in their manufacture and decoration. We then consider modes of viewing, attempting to establish an individual's relationship with, and response to, these miniature hunchbacks, based largely on how and where they would have been displayed. Lastly, we explore some of the motives underlying the miniaturization of the hunchback, suggesting that this was part of a desire to tame and domesticate, and thus normalize, the Other. More generally, this chapter will demonstrate that miniature works of art, as objects often intended for private viewing within a domestic setting, offer access to personal habits of viewing ancient art, allowing us to tap the artistic preferences of non-elite, perhaps even 'ordinary' citizens of the ancient world.[2]

Contextualizing the miniature, contextualizing the hunchback

The study of ancient art has been built upon a hierarchy that sets monumental above miniature, 'major' arts above 'minor' arts and original above copy, all of which are fundamentally connected. Monumental, public sculpture has typically been the focus of art-historical debate on the production and reception of art in antiquity. Miniature, private objects have thus held a secondary, inferior position. The miniature – and indeed the processes and implications of miniaturization – has thus been marginalized in discussions on the artistic repertoire of the ancient past resulting in a limited view of the dynamics that were involved in the conception, production and display of ancient art.[3]

The basis of this hierarchy lies in the content and context of the miniature. Beginning in the Hellenistic period, and continuing well into the Roman period, there developed a trend of representing the underclass of the population (e.g. slaves, foreigners, the ugly, the deformed; all of those marginalized by society) in a miniature format. Of course, there do survive (just under) life-size representations of such unsavoury types as the hermaphrodite, the drunken old woman or the poor, emaciated man, to name just a few, just as there are 'noble' subjects rendered in miniature; however, the former group is much more limited in quantity and quality, and the latter group are often understood as 'copies', interesting only in so far as they refer to large-scale sculptures rather than as objects of art in their own right. There thus seems to be a distinct contrast in the ancient sculptural oeuvre: the body beautiful is lauded in large-scale sculpture and the grotesque body is demoted to small-scale sculpture. This contrast raises the question: how did the ancients perceive the difference in size between subjects and were they predisposed to see them in a certain way or view them in a specific context?

In 1961 Bieber observed that genre or 'lowly' subject matter 'by its very nature lends itself better to small than to monumental size' (Bieber 1961: 95). Thirty years later Bartman noted that 'minor size would seem to be equated with minor social status' (Bartman, *Miniature*, 168). Numerous scholars have attempted to explain and justify this phenomenon. Smith has suggested that 'smaller size might assuage any sense of impropriety at the representation of such lowly subjects in fine statues' (Smith 1991: 137),[4] while Zanker has suggested that 'the execution and medium at least in part ennoble[d] their lowly subjects, engaged in their day to day but still, in their own way, heroic struggles' (Zanker 2004: 138). Thus, given these two modes of scale in ancient sculpture, and how they were applied to various subjects, scholars have very often dismissed the importance of small-scale sculpture, and the miniature hunchback in particular.

To date, representations of the hunchback have been studied in the context of the grotesque. As 'lowly' subject matter, grotesques on the whole have been characterized as 'inferior art'. Indeed, in 1903 Wace asserted that all bronze grotesques (which many of the hunchbacks catalogued are) lacked fine modelling and were often very coarse and rough in execution (Wace, *Grotesques*). This sentiment has become so engrained as to prejudice the opinion of successive scholars studying these representations as a group, rather than as individual types.[5] Notwithstanding this sweeping judgement among scholars of the inferiority of grotesque sculpture in technical execution, a look at the details of the iconography of the corpus of hunchbacks – in particular, the range of materials from which they are produced, the method of their manufacture, and their decoration – reveals a high quality in workmanship and decorative detail. In fact, through an analysis of the hunchback we can re-frame the importance of the miniature – and, indeed, the grotesque body – in a way that heretofore has been summarily dismissed.

Small is beautiful too: the miniature hunchback

A look at the corpus of miniature hunchbacks suggests that at least some representations of the grotesque Other were esteemed for their aesthetic qualities and admired as works of art. Indeed, the range of materials used in the production of the hunchback and the technical virtuosity of their execution seems to have been cause for visual admiration and tactile enticement, thus contributing greatly to their appeal.

Miniature hunchbacks were produced using a range of materials: out of the fifty miniatures catalogued, over half are produced in bronze, a quarter in terracotta, and one in ivory. Those produced in bronze range little in quality, and are, on the whole, carefully fashioned and finely detailed.[6] There are several bronze examples that exhibit exceptional craftsmanship and detail while only a very limited number seem to have been coarsely moulded with little delineation of features. Most representations of the hunchback lie between these two extremes, often delicately rendered, especially in their facial features, which are sometimes depicted in portrait style, and in their anatomical features, especially their humps. The majority of the bronzes are solid cast with the extremities, such as the arms and legs, made separately for attachment (for example, cat. nos **8**, **9** and **33**), which can explain why these parts are so often now missing. The use of separately cast parts for such tiny figures suggests that they must have represented a substantial investment in production time and cost.

In contrast to the solid-cast bronze hunchbacks are a small number that were hollow-cast, which is revealed by small vent holes on the surface; for example, a vent hole is visible on the tunic hanging over the upper left thigh of the hunchback now in the Walters Art Gallery in Baltimore (cat. no. **9**). A number of hollow-cast bronzes reveal a great deal of surface working after casting, for example the facial features, drapery folds and other surfaces are often deeply carved, abraded and faceted. The addition of details to these bronzes after casting is rendered by incision; this is particularly noticeable in the delineation of the hair, where curved lines and dots indicate long and short hair respectively; see, again, the hunchback now in the Walters Art Gallery in Baltimore (cat. no. **9**). Some representations were also inlaid with various precious metals and alloys; four (cat. nos **8**, **9**, **12** and **33**) had various parts, such as the eyes or teeth, inlaid with silver.

A number of the bronze representations in the corpus exhibit extraordinary artistic sophistication and exceptional workmanship. The hunchback now in the Metropolitan Museum of Art in New York (cat. no. **8**) is perhaps the most ornate surviving miniature hunchback produced in bronze and thus warrants a description here. Contested in its date, the statuette is reported to have been discovered on the Esquiline hill in Rome in 1727.[7] The hunchback wears a short tunic that is stitched outside on the right sleeve, buttoned down on the left sleeve and open at the left side. The bottom of the tunic has a fringed border rendered by short vertical incisions. Both hump and phallus are clearly indicated through the thick fabric. The figure also wears thong sandals with one strap running between the first two toes, another around the ankle and tied in a knot at the front and a third running between the sole and the ankle strap. The hair of the hunchback is rendered in two ways: across the top of the head, the hair is formed by sheets of foil, made of copper alloy with an admixture of silver, laid in sections over the surface; around the inlay, curved incisions are used to indicate the short strands of hair, and the hairline recedes on each side of the forehead. The whites of his eyes and his two protruding teeth are silver and the little buttons on the sleeves of his tunic are made of the same copper–silver alloy as the hair. This representation has been praised by numerous scholars because of its artistic erudition. Richter states, 'The execution is excellent; it is both careful and spirited ... moreover, technically, this figure illustrates the extreme care with which some ancient bronzes were worked and decorated' (Richter 1913: 149). Catalogued in *The Gods Delight*, edited by Kozloff and Mitten, the figure is described as 'created with artistry of extraordinary sophistication,' and 'understood as a fine miniature' (Kozloff and Mitten 1988: 165–6).

The hunchback now in the Museum für Kunst und Gewerbe in Hamburg (cat. no. **33**) also ranks as one of the most extraordinary bronzes in the corpus. Of unknown provenance, the figure is dated to the mid third century BCE based on style. The hunchback sits with his legs spread symmetrically and crossed at the ankles. His head is tilted downward and he appears with a sullen and dismal expression. He is missing his right foot and arm, and his neck is cracked, though this does not seem to have altered the intentionally sideways position of the head. The left foot, along with part of the thigh, is not in its original position, but rather twisted slightly upwards. His missing right arm most likely curved with the hand near the right knee, or perhaps rested on the floor near the right side of his bottom or thigh (Jantzen 1958). Notably, the figure grasps the glans of his extraordinarily large penis with his left hand, masturbating (more on this below and in Chapter 3). The eyes and the bared teeth between the lips are inlayed with silver. The figure's careful detailing and quality, with lean and atrophied limbs, hooked nose, ridged, dorsal 'fin'-type hump and tragic facial expression lend to his appeal and admiration; indeed, this figure is hailed as one of the few 'masterpieces' of Hellenistic statuettes.[8] Fowler states that 'this exquisite little bronze' is 'among the most moving and most lovingly made of all the hunchbacks,' whose expression is 'simply heart-rending' (Fowler 1989: 67–9).

Not all of the bronze hunchbacks catalogued are on a par with those just described. At times this is due to the extreme surface damage which some of these statuettes have suffered from 'bronze disease', chloride corrosion caused by contamination from prolonged exposure to water or dirt in burial. Often, it is difficult to determine whether the hunchback is simply crudely fashioned or excessively eroded. An example is the hunchback now in the Wadsworth Atheneum in Connecticut (cat. no. **35**). The statuette was reportedly discovered in Alexandria (although its exact archaeological findspot is unknown) and has been dated to the second century BCE. The statuette depicts a hunchback in the pose of a Spinario: seated on a rock, stooped over with his right leg crossed over the left, attempting to extract a thorn from his right foot. He is nude except for a pointed cap, has thin, elongated limbs and appears to be emaciated. It is difficult to determine whether the figure was coarsely modelled or has suffered excessive corrosion: both the feet and hands have virtually no delineation of individual toes or fingers, except the finger and thumb of the left hand which pull the thorn from his foot. Even the hunchback's hump is roughly rendered, although its angular form, protruding outward and upward, is, nevertheless, visible. This hunchback, however, appears to be the anomaly within the group. Overall, the corpus of miniature bronze hunchbacks reveals careful workmanship and fine detailing.

The terracotta examples of hunchbacks are of lower quality than the bronzes; however, when compared to other terracotta grotesques the level of quality with which the hunchback was produced seems to have been standard.[9] Of the fifteen miniature terracottas catalogued in the corpus, there is little range in quality; most are of an intermediate level, neither exceptionally nor poorly crafted or detailed. A number of these representations are significantly fragmented, surviving only in busts or torsos (cat. nos **49**, **51–5**), thus compromising their analysis here. The majority of these representations are hollow and were assembled from separately made parts. All are moulded on the back, owing to the fact that the hump is the prominent feature on display. Virtually all have hand-modelled facial features. Traces of paint are still visible on a few representations: cat. no. **10** shows traces of red paint on the garment; cat. no. **30** shows traces of a white slip on the body and red paint on the grapes he carries; cat. no. **38** shows traces of red paint on the face and body; and cat. no. **52** shows traces of a white slip and dark red paint on the body; presumably many others would also have had some colouring too. The painting of these figures was surely intended to heighten their aesthetic appeal by adding contrast to the monochrome terracotta, similar to the contrast created by the inlay of various precious metals on the bronzes discussed above. Thus, although produced in a less costly material, these terracotta hunchbacks also reveal a level of care and aestheticism.

The single ivory hunchback now in the British Museum in London (cat. no. **40**) far surpasses in quality many of the other miniature hunchback representations. Although the provenance of this hunchback is unknown, it is assumed to be Egyptian in origin based on its style, although it was reportedly discovered in Italy. This hunchback has been described as 'one of the most haunting works in the entire repertoire of grotesques'.[10] The hunchback is represented seated on a pedestal, holding one knee to the chest and placing the other on the ground with his left hand resting on his left knee and his right arm hanging loosely by his side. His head is large and sunken into his shoulders. He has thin limbs, a protruding pigeon chest, close-cropped hair rendered by small dotted incisions, large ears and a furrowed forehead. The body of the hunchback was carved whole from a single elephant tusk, the pedestal was carved separately, but both are carefully worked and exceptionally detailed, due in part to the intrinsic hardness of the material. We have here a deformed hunchback rendered in a highly exotic and luxurious material, belonging to a series of hunchbacks, which, as we have just demonstrated, are predominantly produced in costly materials, thus revealing that there was a high price afforded to such a 'lowly' or 'insignificant' subject.

The high-quality production of many extant hunchback miniatures suggests that these representations were frequently manufactured to high standards and thus valued as objects of art worthy of display. Although it is difficult to determine the economic and social status of the patron who would have owned a particular miniature hunchback, it seems clear from the variety of materials used and manufacturing standards that these representations appealed to a wide range of patrons, transcending the boundaries of social class and status. Those miniatures at the higher end of the cost spectrum, made of bronze or ivory, with elaborate detail and inlays of silver and various alloys, were likely prized collectors' items owned by wealthy patrons. In contrast, those miniatures at the lower end of the cost spectrum, especially the painted terracottas, would likely have belonged to the non-elite members of society, providing affordable alternatives.

The evident aesthetic appeal of the miniature hunchback raises the questions: where were these (potentially costly) statuettes displayed, for whom and for what purpose? And, moreover, did the aesthetic value of the hunchback complement its function and meaning?

At home with the miniature: displaying the hunchback

The high quality of workmanship with which much of the corpus of hunchbacks was created suggests that some of these representations could surely have been decorative or ornamental, exhibited for personal enjoyment within a private context. The lack of literary evidence regarding the production and display of these representations, however, combined with the fact that many are of unknown provenance, makes determining their display context problematic, but not completely hopeless. We shall examine those (few) representations of the miniature hunchback for which a context is known and reliable, comparing these with other representations of the Other, also of known provenance, as well as examining the broader decorative displays of the ancient miniature, so as to consider some of the reasons for the hunchback's appeal.

As outlined in Chapter 1, the lack of provenance for the majority of hunchback representations results largely from their discovery during uncontrolled archaeological excavations. Out of the fifty-five representations catalogued, twenty-nine have a general provenance recorded.[11] Of these twenty-nine, only seven have a secure archaeological context; however, the exact location within these areas nevertheless remains uncertain. Of the seven, only three comprise miniature statuettes; still, all but one of the seven reveal that at least one possible display context for the hunchback in the Hellenistic and Roman periods was in domestic spaces.[12]

The three miniature statuettes with known provenance have all been recovered from the Roman provinces and two out of the three from villa sites: cat. no. **18** depicts a hunchback playing an instrument – it was found in the Hahnentor area in Cologne; cat. no. **23** depicts a hunchback carrying a cockerel and *lagynos* – it was found in a villa under the Rue du Vieux Marché aux

Vins in Strasbourg; and cat. no. **37** depicts a hunchback holding a string or leather thong to infibulate his penis – it was found in a Roman villa near Herbrechtingen in Stuttgart. All three of the statuettes are made of bronze and are remarkably small, standing, on average, less than ten centimetres high. Other bronze miniatures from the provinces, of comparative style and scale, though of varied provenance, have been thoroughly studied; these are believed to have belonged to Roman soldiers stationed in the provincial outposts and have been attributed a votive or talismanic function.[13] Although we cannot, based on our limited data, assert that the miniature hunchback found in the provinces was a keepsake of the imperial soldier, we may speculate a similar talismanic function, given comparative evidence from elsewhere across the Empire: indeed, it is likely that these statuettes reflect a particularly popular taste for the hunchback as apotropaic talisman or good luck charm, a theme we shall explore in detail in the next chapter.

The rest of the miniature hunchbacks catalogued are without secure provenance. However, given the domestic context of the two statuettes just mentioned, and, additionally, the wall painting (cat. no. **16**), mosaic pavement (cat. no. **17**), bronze vase (cat. no. **20**) and bronze mirror (cat. no. **41**) in the corpus, it seems likely that a domestic setting was at least one, if not *the* principal display context for the miniature hunchback, too. In fact, recent archaeological excavations have recovered an abundance of miniatures, including grotesques, from domestic spaces in Hellenistic Delos, Pergamon and Priene and Roman Pompeii and surrounding areas.[14] Miniature works of art were particularly popular in the private sphere, offering a personal viewing experience that differed significantly from that created by large-scale and monumental works of art set in the public sphere.[15] As summarized by Bartman in her seminal work *Ancient Sculptural Copies in Miniature*, the miniature was highly versatile and could be displayed in a diverse array of decorative design layouts, both indoors, as eye-catching display pieces set atop tables and pedestals or in architectural niches, and outdoors, in a garden as part of the greenery or as a decorative fountain ornament.[16] As such, the miniature was more readily accessible to a viewer, in both visual and tactile ways, and this inevitably contributed to a range of personal interactions and responses. Moreover, a domestic setting for these representations feeds into the underlying motivation for the miniaturization of the hunchback: a desire to tame and domesticate, and thus normalize, the Other, a point upon which I shall elaborate further later.

Miniature representations of the hunchback range in size and height, from 5.1 centimetres to 19.0 centimetres, with an average height of 8.9 centimetres. Their small size has everything to do with their poses: the hunchback is smallest when crouching in a near-foetal position with his head lowered, or, measuring slightly larger, seated on a rock or riding an animal; he is largest when standing fully erect. The poses of the hunchback reveal that the vast majority of these representations would have required some kind of base or pediment upon which the sculpture was mounted, which in turn reveals that these statuettes would have been placed *upon something* for display. Only six representations of the hunchback (cat. nos **5**, **15**, **38**, **45**, **48** and **49**) are equipped with suspension holes or loops, indicating that these hunchbacks were meant to be hung, either from the body or from a building.

The first compositional group, of the hunchback standing or stooping, reveals that at least twenty-one of the thirty-one would have required bases (see cat. nos **2**, **5**, **7**, **8–13**, **18** and **21–31**). Although none of these hunchbacks survive with their original bases, several show markings on the feet indicating they were once attached *to something*. The bases, now often reconstructed for museum display, would have been necessary to keep the hunchback balanced and upright while walking or dancing. Comparative evidence from Priene, where terracotta statuettes from an urban domestic context reveal the use of ledges and niches for display, offers a glimpse of the possible display contexts for the hunchback; but here we must exercise caution: many of the Priene statuettes were drilled with holes to keep them secure, but none of the hunchbacks show signs of similar precautionary measures.[17]

Based on extant evidence, Bartman has documented that tables of either wood, bronze or marble were the most popular form of display support for miniature sculpture; although no archaeological evidence supports this with specific reference to the hunchback, a table would have indeed offered the best views of the miniature hunchback. Tables would have attracted a viewer's attention, first, on account of the fact that they would have raised the miniature hunchback to approximately eye level, and second, through the rich contrast of material, colour and texture when combined with hunchbacks of gilt bronze or painted terracotta.[18] Likewise, pedestals of marble, and other, less imposing pieces of furniture made of different materials (e.g. wood), would have also served as suitable display supports, highlighting the aesthetic character of the miniature hunchback. Moreover, these types of displays allowed the miniature hunchback to be easily examined at various angles – not only at eye level, but literally at hand's reach, suggesting that the hunchback was not just to be *looked at*, but to be picked up, held in one's hand and touched.

By contrast, only two representations of the standing or stooping hunchback are equipped with suspension holes or loops, indicating that they were meant to be hung (cat. nos **5** and **15**). Given their size and symbolism, which will be discussed further below and in the next chapter, it seems that these hunchbacks served as hanging decorations in an indoor architectural setting. As architectural decorations, these hanging hunchbacks might have been less physically accessible to a viewer, indeed perhaps completely out of hand's reach, but the desire to touch them would nevertheless have been present, with viewers being able to imagine their implicit tactility.

The second compositional group, of the hunchback seated or crouching, reveals that six of the sixteen survive on their original bases (see cat. nos **34**, **35**, **40**, **42**, **46**, and **47**). The hunchback now in the Antikensammlung in Berlin (cat. no. **34**) and the hunchback in the Wadsworth Atheneum in Connecticut (cat. no. **35**) sit on rocks, and it is likely that the hunchback in the Museum für Kunst und Gewerbe in Hamburg (cat. no. **33**) was also seated on a rock since its pose is similar.[19] The hunchback now in the de Young Memorial Museum in San Francisco (cat. no. **46**) and the hunchback in the National Archaeological Museum in Athens (cat. no. **47**) ride a donkey or a goat and it is likely that another hunchback in the Antikensammlung in Berlin (cat. no. **44**) was also seated on an animal, given its similar pose. Both of these types of bases suggest a rustic, outdoor setting, which, as comparative evidence from Pompeii and elsewhere shows, was well suited as garden decoration.[20] Indeed, the use of natural landscapes (e.g. rocks) as support for figural representation was fairly common in ancient gardens; several examples of Others will here be examined for comparative analysis with the hunchback.

Representations of the sleeping hermaphrodite were often displayed in an outdoor environment, usually in the garden area of a public (bath) complex or private residence. Depicted resting upon a rocky outcropping, the sleeping hermaphrodite was predominantly sculpted in just under life-size format, but (at least) one miniature hermaphrodite of the sleeping *anasyromenos* type survives from the House of Octavius Quartio (II, 2, 2) in Pompeii (Figure 5).[21] Meauring c. 75 centimetres long, the hermaphrodite is depicted reclining on its back upon a partially preserved rock, partly covered by drapery but with genitals and breasts clearly exposed.[22] The statue was placed against the southern wall of the lower garden, emerging, as it were, from the foliage. Both Tronchin and von Stackelberg have thoroughly analysed the sculptural programme of the House and its eclectic style.[23] Concerning the hermaphrodite's display in the garden, Tronchin asserts that this served multiple functions: it 'alludes to the rural aspect of Hermaphroditus', 'it underscores the myth of Hermaphroditus's origin, which takes place in bucolic surroundings', and finally, its positioning in an out-of-the-way part of the garden 'served as a titillating surprise to the more adventurous guests' (Tronchin 2011: 40). For von Stackelberg the hermaphrodite was more than simply titillating: it cautioned those most daring guests of the 'dangers of encounters between self and other' (von Stackelberg 2009: 125). As the *only* confirmed piece of statuary in the last and largest of four gardens in the House of Octavius Quartio, the

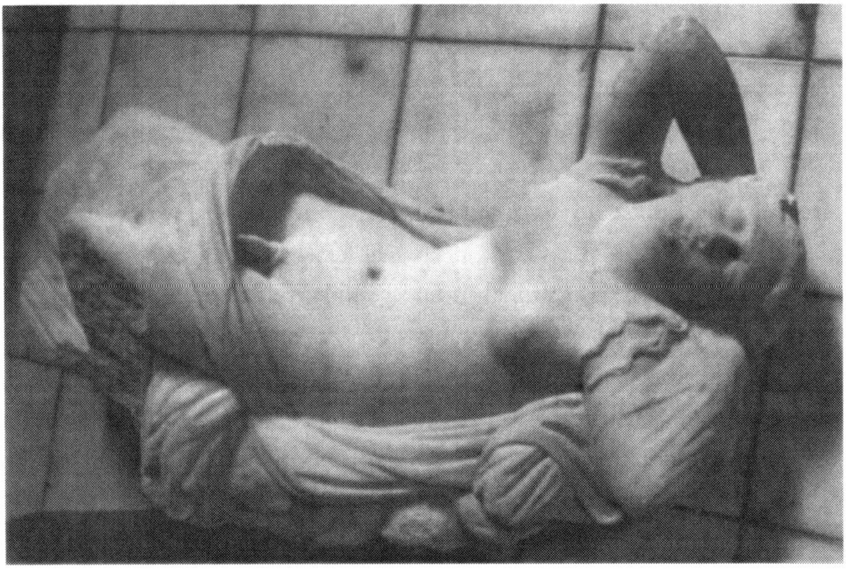

Figure 5 Marble statuette of a sleeping hermaphrodite, c. first century CE. From the lower garden of the House of Octavius Quartio (II, 2, 2) in Pompeii, now Soprintendenza Archeologica di Pompei, 3021.

statue seems to have been purposefully installed to emphasize the landscape of anOther world, to which the hermaphrodite aptly belonged; but this other world had been groomed by design, signifying that the natural world had been conquered and tamed, and so too, the hermaphrodite.

Representations of the Spinario were also suited to an outdoor environment, unsurprising given that the type is inextricably linked with the natural, rural world.[24] The near-life-size (c. 76 centimetres) marble statue of an 'idealized' Spinario now in the British Museum served as an important garden fixture: the rock upon which the boy sits is fitted with holes to accommodate a pipe and reveals evidence of wear from running water, indicating that it functioned as a fountain.[25] Though its context is insecure, the hunchback Spinario now in the Wadsworth Atheneum in Connecticut (cat. no. **35**) perhaps formed part of a fountain, which would explain the excessive degree of corrosion, caused by prolonged exposure to water. Less is known about the display setting of the miniature peasant Spinario now in the Antikensammlung in Berlin, since it was found among a hoard of other terracotta sculptures in an architecturally nondescript room of House 33 in Priene.[26] The miniature versions of the Spinario, both ugly in appearance and uncivilized in their behaviour, parody the idealized type: as Masséglia notes, the peasant Spinario reflects the coarse rustic reality of a low-status labourer, whereas the idealized Spinario reflects the romanticized, Arcadian countryside of the elite.[27]

Like the standing figures above, the tactile qualities of the seated hunchback, – the rocky base and ridged hump – encouraged a viewer to pick up the hunchback and hold it close for inspection. Perhaps there would have been some incentive for a viewer to pick up the hunchback Spinario, whether in a real or imagined way, and examine the thorn in his foot, too; a viewer might thereafter be careful of where he or she treads in the garden so as to not suffer the same annoyance. Like the hermaphrodite, the placement of the hunchback in a garden could be used to emphasize the landscape of anOther world, the taming of that world and, by extension, the taming of the hunchback.

The seated or crouching hunchback is elsewhere represented explicitly in an outdoor setting: the decoration of a bronze mirror in the corpus (cat. no. **41**), which will be thoroughly described and analysed in the next chapter, depicts a lone, ithyphallic hunchback kneeling on the ground, surrounded by flora and birds. It is interesting that such an outdoor scene should decorate an indoor object, and that the 'ugly' hunchback appears on an object used for adornment, where beauty is reflected and/or created. This not only points to the hunchback's role as apotropaic talisman (i.e. protection against envy directed at beauty), but, moreover, his domestication: the un/tamed Other represented outdoors is (to be) fully tamed when brought indoors.

Viewing and touching the hunchback: does size matter?

The miniature size of the hunchback, the tactility implicit in its overall form, and the settings of its display would have positively invited a viewer to physically engage with the statuette and to tactilely explore the body of the hunchback. Indeed, not to touch the hump of the hunchback would be to miss a great deal of its attraction – the smooth, ridged or angular hump protruding from the figure's back was *the* point of focus, tempting a viewer to rub the hunchback's hump. The hunchback thus encouraged viewer integration, creating an intimacy between viewer and statuette: the viewer picked up the hunchback to hold it in his or her hands, *feeling* its contours and moving it around in order to *see* it from every angle.[28] Some of the smallest of hunchback statuettes could surely even have been secreted away on one's person for private delectation.

In this way, these miniature statuettes allowed a viewer the opportunity to (get to) know the body of the hunchback. Because the hunchback could be viewed up close and from all angles, the oddity of his body became a source of contemplation, putting the hunchback, as it were, under the microscope. A viewer was given permission to look at and touch the body of the hunchback with impunity, safe from reprisal, risk or judgement. But in feeling its contours, essentially petting the hunchback, a viewer effectively dehumanized him, turning the hunchback from a man into a thing; a creature whose physicality as a man was mitigated by his miniature size.

In contrast to the miniatures hitherto discussed, only one large-scale sculpture of a hunchback survives: the hunchback now in the Villa Albani-Torlonia (cat. no. **32**). This statue is not only anomalous in the corpus of hunchbacks because of its size, but also because of its context: it is the only representation of a hunchback to have decorated a monumental, public space – it was found in the Baths of Caracalla in Rome. Remarkably, it seems that even in large scale, and even when displayed in a public setting, the hunchback's appeal lay in its implicit tactility and the invitation to touch him: this hunchback provides irrefutable evidence that viewers rubbed the hunchback's hump.[29]

Only the upper torso of this white, fine-grained Luna marble hunchback survives, measuring 56 centimetres high. Both the arms below the shoulders and the legs above the thighs are missing; we cannot therefore determine the full height of the original statue, or its exact pose; however, given the hunchback's forward bent position, and comparison with other miniatures in the corpus similarly represented, it is likely that this hunchback was originally seated. His seated position makes most sense if displayed on a low base, at an equal, or lower, level to passers-by, for the simple reason that the details of his fine representation can be appreciated only if a viewer is standing and looking directly at this hunchback.

The hunchback's body is unnaturally proportioned: his head is excessively large, measuring 27 centimetres, while the entire upper torso measures only 29 centimetres. These dimensions, along with the stunted torso and protruding chest box, give the impression of a dwarf-life physical appearance. The hunchback was also originally endowed with a semi-erect penis (as evidenced in Figure 6), though this was removed and covered by a fig leaf during restorations of the eighteenth century.[30]

The hunchback's deformed body is strikingly juxtaposed with a remarkably handsome, portrait head. The hunchback has a full head of short, thick, curly hair, and wears a full, trimmed beard accompanied by a trimmed lip moustache. He has oval eyes, the irises of which have been drilled, a strong aquiline nose, and thin lips. His head is angled to the right and he gazes upward with slightly furrowed brows, revealing a calm expression of quiet contemplation and reflection. This is not the kind of head one would expect to go with this deformed body, particularly given that the vast majority of hunchbacks in the corpus are depicted with generic, sometimes grotesque, facial features, but the oddity of this disjunction was intentional.[31]

This hunchback was found in the Baths of Caracalla in Rome, although his exact display setting in the Baths is unknown. I have argued elsewhere, based on the decorative programme of the Baths, that the sculpture was likely displayed in one of the Baths' outdoor garden areas, seated upon a (rocky?) base

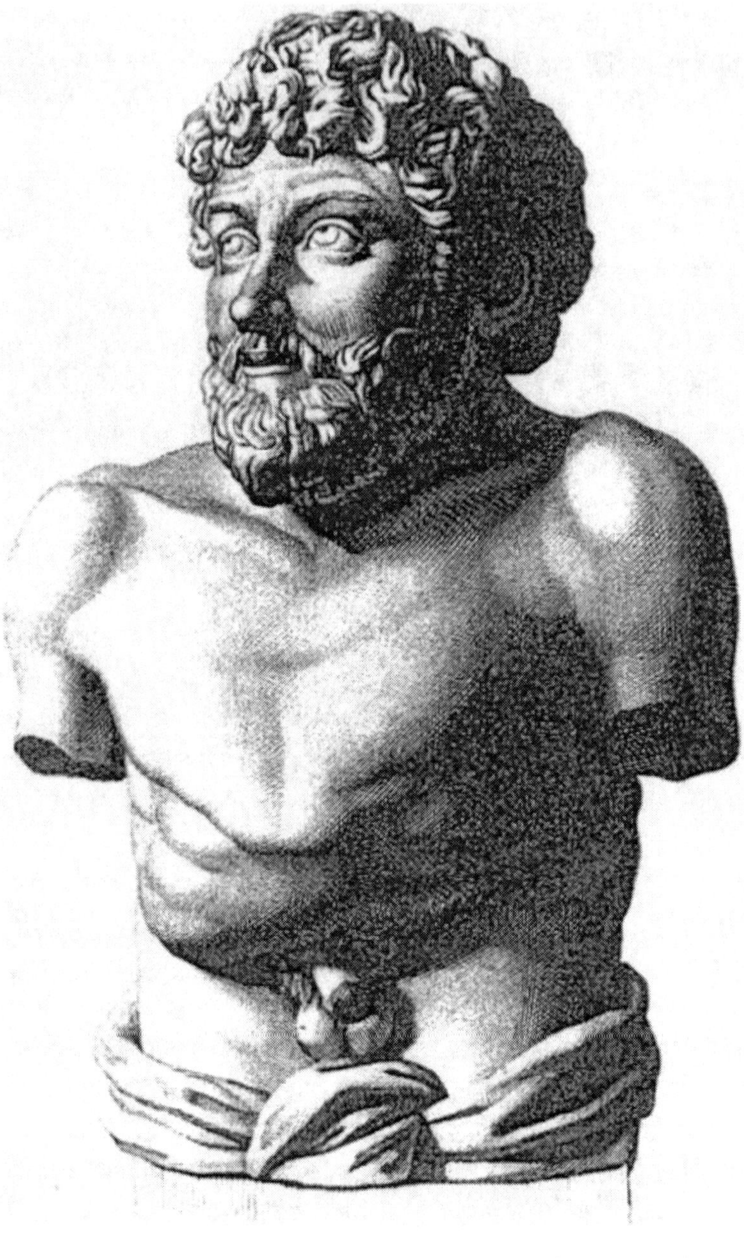

Figure 6 Engraving of the hunchback in the Villa Albani-Torlonia, Rome (cat. no. 32), showing the hunchback as ithyphallic.

set at ground level so as to be at an equal, or lower, height to passers-by (Trentin 2009: 146). Viewing this sculpture fully in the round would have elicited a wide range of responses from a viewer; indeed this seems to have been the function of the hunchback, and many other sculptures in the Baths of Caracalla: the sculptures manoeuvre a spectator's viewing experience through their treatment of front and back, making the viewer the 'dupe' of their programmatic character, shocking and surprising viewers in unexpected ways.[32]

From whichever angle the hunchback is approached, front or back, the sculpture is designed to manipulate a spectator's viewing experience so as to generate a strong response. Approaching this sculpture from the rear puts the hump of the hunchback on display and makes his identity immediately recognizable. Here we must ask: would a viewer have been compelled (and indeed permitted) to touch this large-scale hunchback in the same way as the miniature hunchback? His context within a public space might suggest a 'no touching allowed' or 'hands-off' rule; however, this hunchback provides the best evidence in the corpus for touching the body of the hunchback, specifically his hump: the eroded state of his hump unequivocally demonstrates that rubbing the hump would have been, at least in part, a source of the sculpture's appeal, especially given that the rest of his body reveals no similar signs of significant wear.[33]

Moving around to the front of the figure, a viewer would be shocked to see such a handsome face on an odd and unnatural body type. The hunchback's handsome face contributes to a tension in viewing: because this hunchback looks like it could be *someone*, a specific individual, the safety of anonymity is absent, thus giving the viewer pause: what does it mean to have just rubbed the hump of this *someone*? The addition of the semi-erect penis further exaggerates this tension. The ithyphallic nature of the hunchback could indicate that he functioned as an apotropaion in the Baths; a place where the dangers of the evil eye were ubiquitous. This feature may have been a source of amusement and incited laughter – part of its apotropaic agency – but this is complicated by the hunchback's remarkably handsome face, once again giving the viewer pause: what does it mean to laugh at this *someone*?

Approaching this sculpture from the front creates an equally confounding viewing experience. A viewer would be unexpectedly confronted with a figure whose head is at odds with his body, thus causing the viewer to ponder the oddity of this disjunction (see above). Moving around to the back of the figure also gives the viewer pause: perhaps wanting to rub the hump, a viewer might now question whether such touching is appropriate; this is not the anonymous miniature hunchback familiar from a private setting (to do with as one pleases), it is *someone* (who *is* it?) adorning a public space.[34]

This hunchback, in its display of a body comprising such disparate features (handsome face, deformed body and erect penis), was surely intended to confound a viewer's expectations. A hunchback is perhaps not the ideal piece of statuary one might expect to find in a bath complex – indeed, it is unusual given the domestic context of the other representations in the corpus – but perhaps this was the point of his display. This hunchback's deformity was not minimized or hidden away; rather it was placed in a grand, public setting for everyone to see and, more importantly, judge. The facial expression of the hunchback, of contemplation and reflection, perhaps encouraged a similar response from a viewer, who, after having examined this figure fully in the round, would have been forced to look at this hunchback anew and thereafter reflect upon their own body and mind and to (re-)consider what quality defined them.

As an object of display, in both small and large scale, in private and public contexts, we must imagine that a range of viewers would have seen and, when permitted, touched the hunchback. These different viewers would presumably have had different viewing experiences, with variances based on gender, age, race, ethnicity and 'ability'. The male, able-bodied, adult Roman citizen would respond differently from a young, male slave of foreign origin, or even an older male citizen suffering from some form of disability on account of his age, such as diminishing vision. Moreover, a female viewer would have responded differently from a male viewer to this male body.

Upon handling the hunchback, a(ny) viewer would have had the eerie and awesome experience of feeling a body unlike their own. But what if that body wasn't *so* different from their own? In viewing and feeling the hunchback, would an ancient viewer have thought about his or her own corporeality and (ab)normality? Inescapably, yes. This was perhaps the greatest appeal of the hunchback, regardless of size: forcing a viewer to question the meaning ascribed to the body of the hunchback, and the Other, and indeed, all body types, however near or far from his or her own. Thus the optic and haptic encounter with the hunchback created a uniquely stimulating (physical, intellectual, perhaps even emotional) viewing experience.

Domesticating the hunchback

What was the motivation for the ubiquitous practice of miniaturizing representations of the Other, and the hunchback in particular? As we have seen, the vast majority of representations of the hunchback survive as miniature statues; these statuettes encouraged viewers to pick them up, to handle them, and to rub them, indeed to have them in hand and in home. This physical dominance suggests an attempt to contain and control the hunchback – to domesticate him.[35]

As a deformed Other, the hunchback symbolized the aberrant and mysterious forces of nature and was thus the object of curiosity and concern. By miniaturizing the hunchback, its unruly nature was, in a sense, brought under control, rendering him non-threatening. The high quality of workmanship and decorative detail of the miniature hunchback gave it a level of care and appreciation that made it almost amiable and endearing. Hellenistic and Roman viewers thus appropriated the hunchback for display, thereby exercising control over the body of the Other. As an object of display, the hunchback offered itself to possession, the possession of its (able-bodied, 'normal'?) viewer; a definitive sign of his domestication.

Not coincidentally, it was during the Hellenistic and Roman periods that representations of deformed Others were widely produced; they are represented chiefly as entertainers, dancing, singing and/or playing music.[36] This is precisely the time when such real-life individuals were becoming popular household slaves among the elite. Their popularity is especially well attested among the Romans, though this fad surely developed from an earlier and well-established tradition of displaying the anomalous body in ancient Greek culture, too. Ancient sources claim that some wealthy Romans prized slaves with unusual physical features and obvious physical deformities. Plutarch states that in Rome the demand for deformed slaves was so great that monster markets (*τῶν τεράτων ἀγορὰν*) emerged where persons who 'have no calves, or who are weasel-armed or who have three eyes or who are ostrich-headed' could be purchased.[37]

Quintilian also claims that deformed slaves were in such demand that some Romans were prepared to pay more for them than for physically perfect ones.[38] These (costly) slaves were prized as entertainers and often put on display to provide amusement.[39]

The role of the hunchback as entertainer is well attested in both the literary and visual records; the former survives largely from the Roman world through (mostly Latin) texts of the imperial period, and is both disturbing and entertaining because of the often unusual and bizarre contexts in which the hunchback appears. Lucian describes a banquet in which a hunchback with an Egyptian accent recites some anapests in time with the clapping of his hands, thus entertaining his guests.[40] Pliny too recounts a story of a wealthy woman, Gegania, who, at a dinner party, had her hunchback slave, Clesippus, perform naked to entertain her guests. Gegania thereafter fell in love with the hunchback, admitting him to her bed and then later giving him a place in her will; a definitive act of domestication.[41] Equally famous is the story recounted in the 'Life of Commodus' in the *Scriptores Historiae Augustae*. As part of a long diatribe against the emperor's monstrous habits, the reader is told that Commodus displayed two misshapen hunchbacks at a private banquet, served on a silver platter and smeared with mustard, thereafter advancing and enriching them.[42] That the hunchbacks are smeared with mustard – physically rubbed to obtain the desired effect – displayed on a silver platter and then, only after this humiliating experience, are promoted and enriched, indicates that the prosperity of the hunchbacks hinges on their debasement; much like Gegania's hunchback slave.

For those who could not afford the exorbitant prices demanded for such real-life curiosities, perhaps owning a representation in miniature was enough; with plenty of options available, these miniatures appealed to a wide range of patrons, from those willing to splurge on the more costly hunchbacks made of bronze and inlaid with precious metals, to those who couldn't, in which case the cheaper terracottas would do. This provided a way of affirming an individual's status and position within the community of elite – or aspiration to membership within it. To own a representation of a hunchback was, as Masséglia notes, an attempt to 'buy into the high end of the entertainment market', for only those with money could afford the real-life hunchback.[43]

The hunchback as entertainer is evidenced in the visual record in a variety of media: six statuettes (cat. nos **11–15** and **24**) depict the hunchback dancing, and two statuettes (cat. nos **18** and **19**) appear to be playing an instrument. Likewise, two miniatures (cat. nos **48** and **49**) function as hanging vases and, on account of their iconography (note, in particular, the ivy wreath worn by cat. no. **48**), have been interpreted as decorative fixtures representing sympotic entertainers or court jesters (Perdrizet 1911: 59–60, no. 96; Giuliani 1987; Barton 1993).

One statuette in the corpus was almost certainly used as a decorative fixture: a bronze hunchback now in the Antikensammlungen in Munich (cat. no. **15**) measuring 8.5 centimetres in height, dating broadly to the late Hellenistic/early Roman period. The hunchback is depicted wearing, rather precariously, a vase on top of his head; the vase is a wine amphora, the handles of which serve as the suspension for his hanging display. The hunchback appears to be in the midst of jumping, likely performing some dance routine. He has elongated, elastic limbs; his left leg is raised and bent at the knee while his right leg hangs loosely and his enormously long penis dangles in between. Masséglia observes that he seems to be kicking his own oversized penis with the heel of his left foot: a dance manoeuvre that may have been quite familiar (Masséglia, *Body Language*). Although the arms are no longer attached, presumably these would have been raised and/or outstretched.[44]

This hunchback effectively breaks into the viewer's space. We might imagine that if this was a real-life hunchback one would have to take a step back, for at any moment a viewer might be hit by a flying arm or leg (or if really unfortunate, some other body part!) or might even find him or herself in the path of a flying vase. The pose of this hunchback was surely intended to provoke laughter – and therefore aided in its use as an apotropaic talisman – but it also served as a tell-tale sign of his profession as an entertainer. As a decorative fixture at the symposium or convivium at which the real-life hunchback may have performed, this statuette would have bestowed festive hilarity while reminding a viewer of his own privileged social status, wealth and good fortune.

Beyond the miniature hunchback, there are other representations in the corpus where we find the hunchback engaged in some kind of performance, for instance the wall painting and mosaic pavement (cat. nos **16** and **17**, respectively) where the hunchback carries rhythm sticks denoting that he is dancing. Perhaps the most compelling piece of evidence for the role of the hunchback as entertainer, and his domestication as such, is his representation on a small bronze vase, also in miniature scale (21 centimetres high), found at a Roman villa in the Rhône Valley, dating to the first century CE (cat. no. **20**; see also Figure 7). This vase is remarkable on account of its overall decorative scheme. The central panel of this vase depicts the scene of a feast. Fillets and an amphora hang from the wall and four dwarfed individuals, all dressed in loincloths and pointed caps, the hallmark of the clowning (and foreign) entertainer, are represented performing various tasks. One of the central characters in this feast is a hunchback playing the double-flute. He stands to the left of a low, three-legged table upon which have been placed three different-shaped vases. To the right of this table another figure appears holding a cup, a ladle and a third unidentified object, as if he were performing some balancing trick. To the far left of the scene a third figure appears dancing with cymbals. To the far right of the scene a fourth figure appears poking the fire of a blaze on top of which is placed an amphora. Although the exact nature of the feast is unknown, the figures themselves have been interpreted as Dionysian revellers, though I am not entirely convinced of this interpretation and opt rather for a more general interpretation that the scene depicts an entertaining troupe.[45] Regardless, it is not coincidence that these four deformed individuals appear on a vessel that would likely have been used at the very feast where such individuals performed.

Interesting also is the scene decorating the neck of this vase and the detailing of the handle. The neck of the vase depicts an Egyptian Nilotic panorama: a naked pygmy wearing only a hat (or helmet of some sort) but armed with a

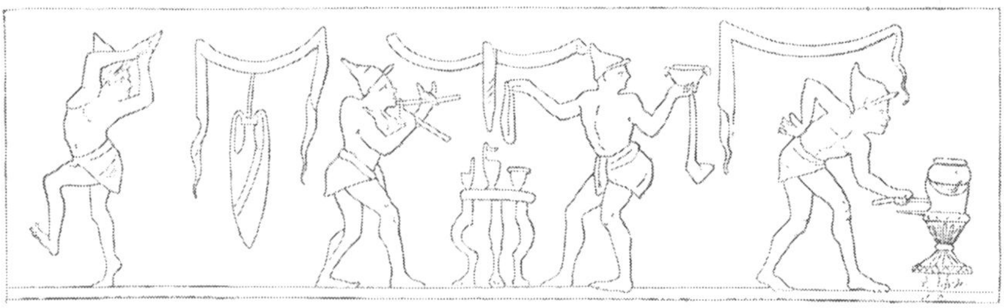

Figure 7 Detail of the central panel of a bronze vase from the Rhône Valley (cat. no. 20), depicting a hunchback as part of an entertaining troupe at a feast.

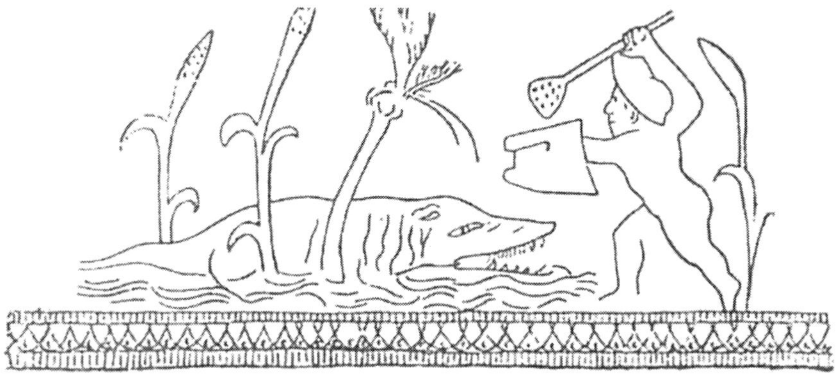

Figure 8 Detail of the neck of a bronze vase from the Rhône Valley (cat. no. 20), depicting a Nilotic scene with an armed pygmy attacking a crocodile.

weapon (stick or sword?) and shield appears ready to attack a large crocodile sitting in a swampy marsh along the Nile (Figure 8). The depiction of pygmies battling crocodiles was particularly popular in Nilotic scenes on wall paintings and mosaic pavements from villa sites and tombs across Italy and the Roman provinces from the first century BC onwards.[46] These paintings bring the Other physically into the domestic sphere, thus appropriating and legitimizing his display. The pairing of the two scenes on the vase seems to illustrate the division between the foreign, uncivilized Other, i.e. the pygmy attacking a crocodile in an outdoor environment, and the tamed, domesticated Other, i.e. the hunchback and the dwarf performing various tasks in an indoor environment, at a feast. This division is accentuated by the handle of the vase, restored in the third century CE. Depicted at one end, aligned with the spout of the vase, is a seated lion; at the other end, aligned with the central panel, is the face of a beautiful woman. The foreign and the familiar are here again to be viewed one against the other.

As an object of considerable worth (being made of bronze and richly decorated) this vase was likely reserved for use at special occasions, the banquet or drinking party. At such occasions there would have been lavish entertainment aimed at impressing the guests: music, dancing, mimes, etc., which may very well have been performed by deformed slaves, like the hunchback or dwarf, depending on the (financial) means of the host. We must also imagine a wide collection of other decorative objects (miniature statuettes, wall paintings and so on) contributing to a viewer's response to this vase and its decoration, and the conversation it might therefore stimulate in context. The vase probably held wine, poured for guests by (deformed?) slave attendants. Physically holding the vase in his or her hand to empty its contents allowed not only the slave be-holder to view its decorative scenes, but the guests as well. These viewers would have responded differently to the scenes illustrated: for guests, the vase reminded them of their privileged status; for slaves, their lowly status. Moreover, in its overall decoration, with its exotic, Egyptianizing theme, the vase reminded both slave and guest of their place in an Empire where conqueror and conquered coexisted in strictly defined hierarchies, thus affirming (but still blurring) the distinction between Self (viewer: conqueror: domesticator) and Other (viewed object: conquered: domesticated).

Thus, the hunchback's position as an entertainer, especially when represented in miniature sculpture, but also as a small-scale relief painting, became symbolic of his domestication. Through the scale, pose and gestures of these hunchbacks, artists strove to contain and control the hunchback, thus allowing him a place among the 'normal'-bodied. But this place was a precarious one, complicated by the division between real life and representation, a theme which will be further explored in Chapter 4.

3

Kai Su? The Hyperphallic Hunchback

A large proportion of representations of the hunchback are depicted as hyperphallic: of the fifty-five representations catalogued, thirty are endowed with large genitals, characterized by a disproportionately long and/or erect penis, known as macrophallic and ithyphallic respectively, which tends to a club shape, having a narrow base and a bulging glans.[1] Looking beyond the hunchback, representations of the Other (e.g. the black African, dwarf, hermaphrodite and satyr, to name just a few) are also often depicted with exaggerated sexual attributes. In contrast, a scan of Greco-Roman visual art reveals that the ideal male (human, heroic or divine) was almost always depicted with improbably small, pert and boyish genitals, characterized by a thin and short penis and a small scrotum.[2] Why did artists choose to represent the Other as hyperphallic and why did consumers want to look at (and possibly touch) these representations?

This chapter will explore the meaning of hyperphallicism in ancient art by deploying detailed analysis of the hyperphallic hunchback. We begin by examining the most widely recognized interpretation for their function: apotropaic charms used to ward off the evil eye of envy.[3] We will focus on ten examples from the corpus that explicitly served such a function (cat. nos **5**, **13–17**, **24**, **33**, **38** and **41**), assessing why the hunchback seems to have been a particularly efficacious character in warding off evil. Then, placing these representations within a wider visual and literary tradition, we will explore other, complementary functions, equally important, but mostly overlooked, for understanding this complex iconography. As we shall see, some of these representations could be erotically charged, that is, sexually stimulating and titillating to certain viewers; this reading is both separate from, and intimately linked to, an apotropaic function.

The hunchback as apotropaion

In ancient Mediterranean culture, as today, the belief in, and thus the need for protection against, the evil eye of envy was widespread.[4] Literary and archaeological evidence suggests that individuals took the precaution of wearing apotropaic charms and applying apotropaic inscriptions and images in areas where the misfortunes of the envious eye were thought to be particularly dangerous. One of the key characteristics of such apotropaia was the exaggeratedly long or erect penis, known as a phallus.[5] Representations of the phallus alone, or of phalluses which take on human forms, or which become the obvious focal point of a human figure, were widely regarded as potent in averting evil. Emphasis on the phallus in representations of Others, especially deformed Others like the hunchback, points to their use as apotropaia.[6] But it was not just the hunchback's phallus that marked him as an apotropaion, it was also his *atopia*, or unbecoming physical appearance; that is, his hump, and the disproportion of his often dwarfed body, and the presence of (caricatured) black African features, which positioned him outside Greco-Roman standards of beauty, thereby eliciting laughter and dispelling evil.[7] Indeed, the body of the hunchback seems to have been widely recognized as particularly efficacious in warding off evil; this is borne out in both the literary and visual records.

Ancient literature provides clear evidence for the body of the hunchback functioning as an apotropaion. Most revealing is an episode in the life of the famous Greek fabulist Aesop who, according to tradition, was of misshapen appearance: he was a flat-nosed, pot-bellied, bow-legged, hunchbacked dwarf with a flat neck and pointed head (Perry 1936: 40).[8] In the surviving texts of the *Life of Aesop* we are told that Aesop was a slave, purchased as a (*προσ*)*βάσκανιον* precisely because of his ugly and deformed appearance.[9] When Aesop is taken home by his master Xanthus, the other (average- to good-looking) slaves explain why their master has invested in such a foul body. In one version of the *Life*, the slaves speak to one another:

> *οἱ δὲ δοῦλοι πρὸς ἑαυτούς . νὴ τὴν Νέμεσιν τί ἐγένετο τω δεσπότῃ τοιοῦτον κακοπινὲς σῶμα ἀγοράσαι; ἄλλος .οἶδας γὰρ διὰ τί αὐτὸν ἠγόρασεν. ἄλλος. Πρὸς τί; ἵνα αὐτὸν προσ-βάσκανον τοῦ σωματεμπορίου ποιήσῃ.*

> The slaves said to themselves: 'By Nemesis, what made our master purchase such a filthy creature?' One of them said, 'Don't you not know why he has bought him?' When he asked why, he replied: 'So that he might employ him as an apotropaeum for the slave-shop.'[10]

In another version of the *Life*, the slaves speak in unison:

> *τί γέγονε τῷ δεσπότῃ, ὅτι τοιοῦτον κακοπινὲς ἠγόρακε σωμάτιον; πλὴν προς βάσκανίαν τοῦ σωματεμπορίου αὐτὸν ὠνήσατο.*
>
> What has become of our master that he has purchased such a filthy creature? It can only be that he has bought him to protect the slave-shop from envious fascination.[11]

The body of the hunchback Aesop seems well suited as an apotropaion in the slave-shop. Other literary and visual sources supplement this account and demonstrate that representations of hunchbacks were used to protect many other types of buildings, too.

Hanging statuettes: the hanging hunchback

Literary sources confirm the use of apotropaia in the form of hanging statuettes, which, like the body of the hunchback Aesop, are somehow strange or misshapen: Pollux of Naucratis, a second-century CE scholar and rhetorician, states that it was customary for blacksmiths to hang *βασκάνια* ('strange' objects) from their furnaces to ward off envy.[12] Likewise, Phrynicus of Bithynia, a second-century CE rhetorician and grammarian, notes that *βασκάνια* ('man-like' creatures departing in some measure from human nature) were hung by craftsmen at their places of work.[13]

Six statuettes in the corpus of hunchbacks (cat. nos **5**, **15**, **38**, **45**, **48** and **49**) are equipped with suspension holes, suggesting that these hunchbacks were meant to be hung, either from the body or from a building. Of these statuettes, three (cat. nos **5**, **15** and **38**) are represented as hyperphallic and functioned as apotropaia.

A terracotta hunchback now in the Antikensammlungen in Munich (cat. no. **5**) was hung by means of the hole drilled through the hump on his back. This hunchback is the largest miniature in the corpus, measuring 19.0 centimetres in height. Given his size, it is unlikely that this hunchback would have been hung from the body – although of unknown provenance, we might imagine instead that he hung in a building (perhaps a slave-shop or blacksmith's shop?). Represented nude and emaciated with his hands loosely clasped on his chest, this hunchback was identified by Sieveking (1930: 19) as an apotropaion; Dunbabin and Dickie (1983: 20–21) demonstrate that he was not simply a charm against envy but an actual physical personification of envy. This hunchback belongs to a group of grotesque figures who represent envy: a character 'wasted with misery, choking on his own bile' (Dunbabin and Dickie 1983: 21).[14] This is a powerful symbol of the hunchback's potency: he can be both a protector against envy and the embodiment of the dangerous enemy against which protection is required.

We have already seen in Chapter 2 that a bronze hunchback also in the Antikensammlung in Berlin (cat. no. **15**) could have functioned as an apotropaion: the exposure of this hunchback's enormously long penis, combined with his 'penis-kicking' pose, was surely intended to provoke laughter, and therefore aided in its use as an apotropaic charm. But the statuette also served as a sympotic decoration, bestowing festive hilarity while reminding a viewer of his own privileged status.

The same is true of the hanging hunchback now in the Louvre (cat. no. **38**). This small terracotta from Smyrna, measuring 7.5 centimetres in height, depicts a dwarfed hunchback endowed with an enormously large (in length and thickness) penis – indeed, it is by far the largest example in the corpus. This overly exaggerated feature alone suggests his role as an apotropaion; this is further confirmed by traces of red paint on his face and body: red was the most powerful apotropaic colour in antiquity, and still to this day in many parts of the world (Dundes 1981: 61, 63). But the hunchback is also depicted with an ivy crown upon his head, and his gaping mouth and facial expression suggest that he is performing: he too is an entertainer and likely served as a sympotic decoration.[15]

Mosaic pavements: the lucky hunchback

Perhaps the best example of the hunchback's use as an apotropaion is demonstrated by a mosaic pavement (cat. no. **17**) that once decorated the main vestibule to the peristyle court in the House of the Evil Eye, a Roman villa in

Jekmejeh, south-west of Antioch, dating to the second century CE.[16] The mosaic, measuring 0.84 metres high by 0.83 metres wide, features a solitary hunchback, dwarfed in corporeal proportion, depicted with pink flesh, dark brown-black hair and eyebrows, and wearing a short, grey and white loincloth that does little to conceal his erect phallus. The hunchback strides towards the left, looking back over his right shoulder, thus directing a viewer's gaze to his prominent hump. He carries in each hand a light brown stick that forks at either end – rhythm sticks that indicate he is dancing.[17] Above the hunchback appears the phrase *καὶ σύ* in black.[18] This cursory phrase has strong apotropaic associations: it may have served as a simple warning to visitors of the villa that whatever ill will or good wishes they felt towards the household were being sent back to them, or it may have served as a prophylactic curse, perhaps translated as 'may you also suffer ill' and understood as spoken by the hunchback and directed at a viewer.[19]

This mosaic was paired with another, marginally bigger, measuring 0.87 metres high by 0.85 metres wide, laid a few feet above, featuring Herakles as a baby strangling the snakes sent by Hera to kill him (Figure 9). Herakles' body is plump and infantile but his head, with dark brown-grey hair and full eyebrows, looks like that of an adult; this contrasts the hunchback who, even as an adult, is represented with a child's dwarfed body.[20] Herakles, like the hunchback, is also depicted with pink flesh, but sits rather than stands. He kneels on his left knee and wears a light brown cloak with yellow highlights, thrown over his shoulder. He holds the head of one snake in his left hand close to his left thigh and the other in his right hand, without looking at either of them; rather, he gazes outside of the mosaic's frame towards the left in the opposite direction to that of the hunchback. As snakes were powerful prophylactic symbols and feature regularly among the creatures that attack the evil eye, Levi has argued this is the first time that the episode of Herakles strangling the snakes was used for an apotropaic purpose (Levi, *Lucky Hunchback*, 230–32). Its apotropaic function would have complemented that of the hunchback mosaic with which it was viewed.

Although these two mosaic panels were discovered in perfect condition, a much larger mosaic pavement, measuring 1.74 metres high by 1.47 metres wide, was laid above them at a later date, the apotropaic function of which is

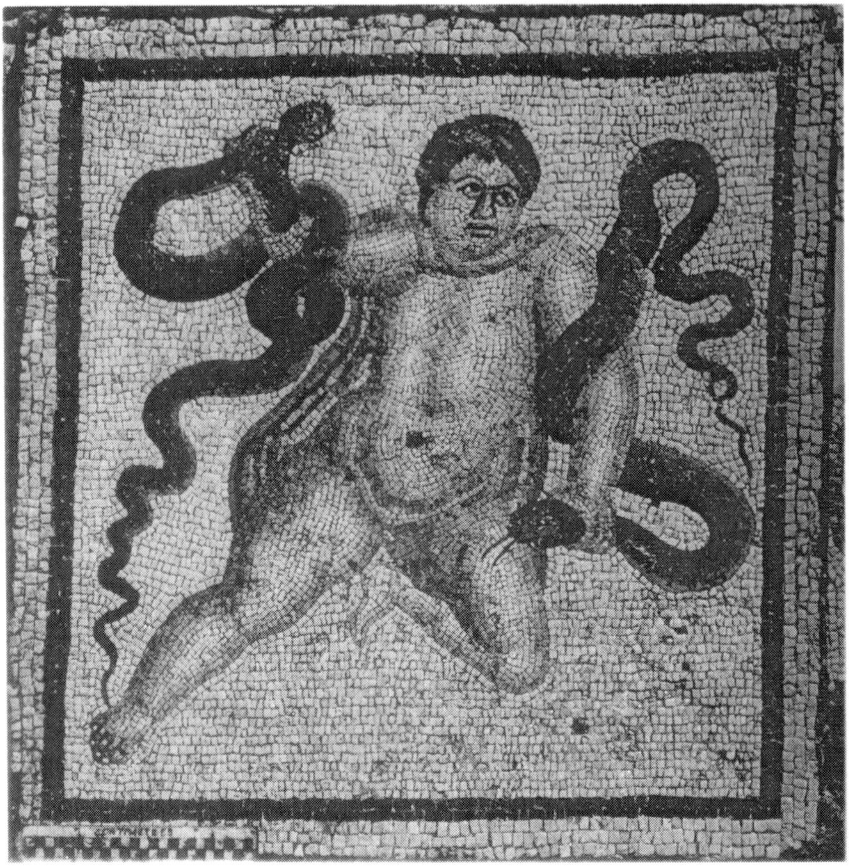

Figure 9 Mosaic pavement depicting baby Herakles strangling snakes, c. second century CE. From the House of the Evil Eye in Jekmejeh near Antioch, now Hatay Archaeology Museum, Antakya, 1026/b.

far more explicit (Figure 10). This mosaic features a large eye (an evil eye) being viciously attacked by various animals and weapons, including a trident and sword, snake and scorpion, dog and panther, and a raven and centipede.[21] To the left of the eye is a dwarf who appears with his back to the eye.[22] He carries rhythm sticks, similar to those carried by the hunchback. The dwarf is endowed with a large phallus, which projects out below his buttocks, stretching towards the eye, as if to attack it too.[23] Above the dwarf, the phrase *καὶ σύ* appears, this time in red; the change in colour is surely intended to strengthen its apotropaic potency.

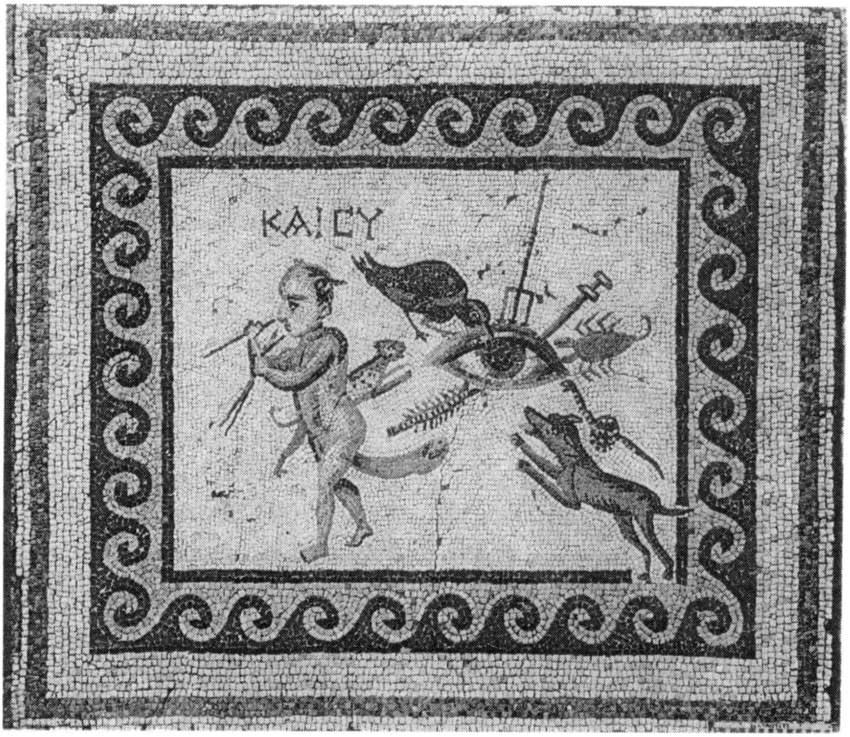

Figure 10 Mosaic pavement depicting an ithyphallic dwarf and the evil eye, c. second century CE. From the House of the Evil Eye in Jekmejeh near Antioch, now Hatay Archaeology Museum, Antakya, 1024.

The association of the phallic dwarf with the evil eye makes the apotropaic function of this mosaic obvious; its shared iconography with the mosaics beneath – the *atopia* of Herakles and the hunchback, the cursory *καὶ σύ* inscription, and the repetition of the snake – confirm their apotropaic function. The owner of this villa was clearly enjoying protection from a number of different apotropaic images: hunchback, deity and dwarf.

In analysing these mosaics, scholars have focused solely on their use as apotropaia, arguing that it was a viewer's laughter at the sight of the dwarf and the hunchback that would have dispelled the evil feared by a viewer (Levi, *Lucky Hunchback*, 225; Clarke 2007: 160). But would laughter have been the only response to these figures? It might have been the anticipated response, and perhaps even the most common response, but it was certainly not the only one; as we saw in the previous chapter, representations of the hunchback worked to confound a viewer's expectations and could elicit a wide range of responses. Like the miniature statuettes, these mosaics engaged a viewer in active viewing. The sheer size of the mosaics and their placement (Figure 11) suggests that a viewer might have to be careful when passing through the vestibule to the peristyle court so as to not step on the hunchback or baby Herakles, although perhaps stomping on the eye in the dwarf mosaic would have been an added protective measure. The high quality of these mosaics, evidenced in their decoration and detailing, would have also demanded that a viewer lean in or crouch down to get the best view of the fine figures depicted; perhaps tracing the outline of the hunchback's hump was equally enticing as rubbing the hump of the hunchback in sculptural form. But even without touching the hunchback, a viewer was compelled to question the meaning ascribed to the body of this figure: the pairing of the hunchback with Herakles is significant in that it places two extremes of appearance, one depiction of physical deformity, the other of physical strength, on the same plane so as to be viewed one against the another.

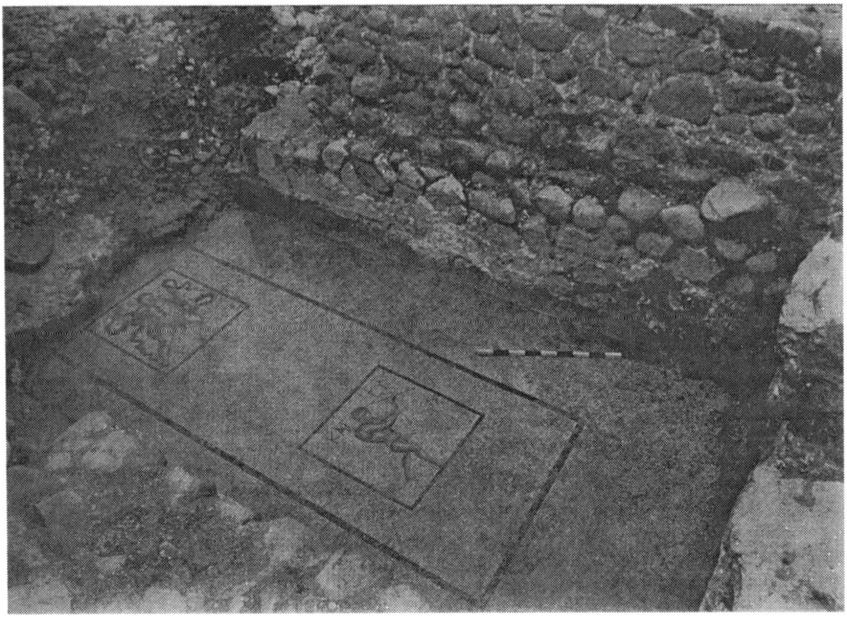

Figure 11 Photograph of the positioning of the hunchback mosaic (cat. no. 17) and baby Herakles mosaic (Figure 9 above) in the vestibule of the 'House of the Evil Eye' in Jekmejeh near Antioch.

The implication of the phrase *καὶ σύ* could perhaps be read outside of its cursory context: translated simply 'and you' it demands that a viewer weigh him/herself against these two extremes, prompting a viewer to consider his/her own (ab/normal) position along a sliding scale of divine and debased.

Miniature statuettes: the 'tuck-for-luck' hunchback

The Antioch mosaics highlight a specific feature that seems to have enhanced the apotropaic power of the Other: the phallus projecting backward, coined by Masséglia as the 'tuck-for-luck' (dancing) pose.[24] The dwarf in the Antioch mosaic is represented with his back turned away from (the gaze of) the eye but his phallus projects backward from beneath his buttocks to directly attack the eye. A number of dwarfs in the form of miniature statuettes are similarly represented. Germaise catalogues at least five such examples, including a dwarf now in the Museum of Fine Arts in Boston depicted with multiple phalluses: an erect phallus projecting forward, an erect phallus (now broken off) projecting beneath his buttocks, and a flaccid phallus attached to the back of his head and drooping over his forehead through which a chain would have been threaded (Figure 12).

Four hunchbacks in the corpus are also represented in the 'tuck-for-luck' pose: cat. nos **13**, **14**, and **24**, and even though his phallus is now broken off, based on his dancing pose and the bulge below his buttocks, it looks as though cat. no. **12** was also depicted in this way. The hunchback now in the Phoenix Gallery of Art in Geneva (cat. no. **13**), of unknown provenance, measures 7.8 centimetres in height and dates to the second century BCE. This nude and emaciated hunchback with protruding chest box is represented dancing. The figure appears to be lifting off, or landing from, a jump: the weight of his body rests on the toes of his left foot and both legs are bent and crossed. Noticeably, the hunchback's large phallus is tucked between his thighs so that it protrudes from beneath his buttocks. Another hunchback, also now in the Phoenix Gallery of Art in Geneva (cat. no. **14**) and of the same date but measuring slightly larger at 8.3 centimetres, is also represented dancing and with his large phallus tucked and protruding from beneath his buttocks. This hunchback is nude and emaciated, but wears a pointed cap held in place by a band, which appears to be decorated (with a diadem?) just above the forehead. He also

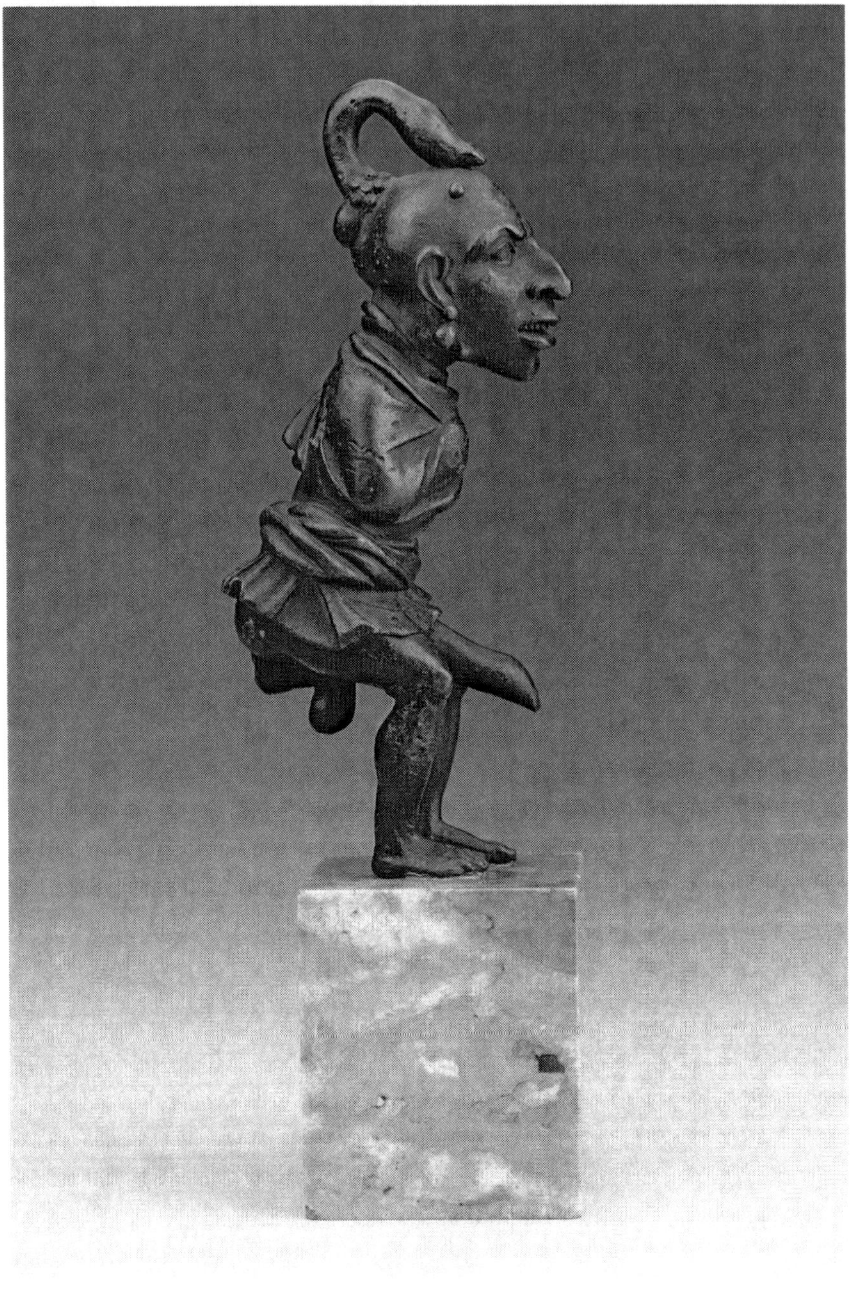

Figure 12 Bronze statuette of an ithyphallic dwarf, c. first century BCE to first century CE. Museum of Fine Arts, Boston, RES.08.32d.

wears a richly decorated band (necklace?) around his neck. Given this hunchback is decked out in finery, perhaps he was intended to explicitly reference the kind of parties where those with money could employ such a distinctive hunchback dancer. The pose of these two hunchbacks and, indeed, everything about their representation – their nudity, emaciated frames and protruding chest boxes – bear similarity to the hunchback now in the British Museum in London (cat. no. **12**), whose phallus is broken off.

Rather different is the hunchback now in the Antikensammlung in Berlin (cat. no. **24**). He is neither emaciated nor does he possess a protruding chest box. This hunchback belongs to the group of hunchbacks catalogued carrying a cockerel and a vase (cat. nos **22–6**), but is anomalous in the group in that although he carries a cockerel, the position of his arm and the shape of the broken object he holds makes it unlikely that he once carried a vase. Also, he is the only hunchback in this grouping represented wearing an ivy wreath and set in the 'tuck-for-luck' pose. It is likely then that this hunchback is represented dancing and that the unidentified object in his left hand is a castanet; he too is an entertainer. But what of the cockerel? The cockerel might be an added apotropaic charm, or, concomitantly, stand as a symbol of fecundity. The cock, as an animal symbolic of male fertility and erotic love, had a long tradition of representation in Greco-Roman art, and may here be used to suggest some kind of erotic association with the hunchback, or the hunchback's use as a charm to boost sexual potency; points upon which I shall elaborate further later.[25]

These four hunchback statuettes seem to have functioned in the same way as the dwarf in the Antioch mosaic: not only is the phallus reproaching evil from behind, but we must imagine that the hump of the hunchback is in some way a powerful weapon against evil, too. Perhaps this was part of the appeal of rubbing the hump of the hunchback – it is used to ward off danger and thus has protective properties. When coupled with the 'tuck-for-luck' pose, the efficacy of the hunchback is even more pronounced.

An Etruscan mirror: the domesticated hunchback

Another example in the corpus provides yet further evidence of the hyperphallic hunchback's use as an apotropaion: a bronze mirror (cat. no. **41**) found in the area of Tarquinia. Although its precise findspot is unknown, the mirror certainly came from one of Tarquinia's many necropoli, in which an abundance of mirrors have been found dating from the mid sixth to the second centuries BCE.[26]

The mirror, measuring 14.1 centimetres high by 13.8 centimetres wide, is engraved, like all Etruscan mirrors, on the reverse, the opposite side of the reflective disc. It was fitted with a rectangular tang to be inserted into a handle, probably of organic material, which has since decayed. The decoration consists of a garland of a continuous ivy-leaf wreath pattern, with large, heart-shaped leaves with stems, surrounding the main medallion design without interruption.[27] The medallion features a naked hunchback, otherwise deformed with a protruding chest box and stumped feet. He is depicted kneeling on the ground with his erect phallus pointing upward between his legs. His right arm is extended horizontally with a bird perched on his right hand. Two additional birds (flying or resting) appear above the hunchback's head facing one another.

Although most Etruscan mirrors with known provenance have been found in tombs, they were certainly not made specifically for the grave, but their secondary setting as a grave good suggests that they provided apotropaic protection both in life *and* in death. Used during the lifetime of the deceased as an object of female adornment, mirrors not only served a utilitarian function, but also had symbolic and magical connotations. The user of the mirror was obviously involved in rituals of (narcissistic) beautification, and thus was especially prone to eliciting the evil eye of envy from spectators. The mirror itself, which was a highly valued item of considerable craftsmanship, in metal-smithing and creative skill and in the incised detail of the figural decoration, thus signified a level of status and wealth, adding yet another layer of potential envy. The user thus took the precaution of ornamenting this mirror with an apotropaic image – an ithyphallic hunchback – to avert evil. As the hunchback does not appear as a stock image for Etruscan mirrors – indeed, no other image of a hunchback has been identified in the corpus of Etruscan mirrors – we can suppose that the owner of this mirror had a specific, personal reason for choosing the hunchback, perhaps believing it offered good luck.

As an apotropaion, the mirror was equally important to its owner beyond their lifetime into their death, since it also functioned as a grave good. Based on analyses of other mirrors found at Tarquinia and other apotropaic tomb imagery found across Italy, we can make some inferences about the mirror's use as an apotropaion in death. Clarke has convincingly argued that representations of dwarfs and pygmies in Nilotic scenes on wall paintings decorating tombs in Italy had an apotropaic function, simultaneously providing protection from evil spirits to the guests of the tomb, and also frightening the evil spirits of death who looked upon these images (Clarke 2007a and 2003, esp. 191–215). As we have already attributed an apotropaic function to the mirror in life, it follows that this apotropaic function continued in death, helping to deflect any harm that might come to the deceased. However, a curious feature of the mirrors found *in situ* at the tombs in Tarquinia is that they were oriented so that the figural scenes were hidden, meaning that the obverse, the reflecting mirror side, was visible. As an apotropaic device, we might expect that the figured representation of the hunchback would be face up (in fact, it may well have been) to avert evil forces and demons. But Carpino (2008: 24–5) and de Grummond (1991: 22) suggest that the 'reflection-death' superstition was more potent: because the obverse both projects and reflects the image of its user it was thus considered a receptacle for the soul of the deceased, helping the soul journey to the afterlife without harm. Thus, a mirror's use to both reflect and deflect images, in life and in death, demonstrates that it was well suited as an apotropaic device. The image of the hunchback as apotropaion on this specific mirror, however, would seem to have been more potent against the living than the dead.

Like the hunchback represented on the mosaic from Jekmejeh, the significance of the hunchback depicted on this mirror goes beyond its apotropaic function. The fact that this ithyphallic hunchback is represented in an idyllic, outdoor landscape, but is depicted on an indoor object of female adornment, and then is brought to the grave, highlights the hunchback's full domestication. His domestication thus allows for a more intimate encounter between viewer and object. Holding the mirror in one's hand – held at arm's length much of the upper body would be in view – enabled the primary be-holder to admire her own reflection. It also allowed secondary viewers (e.g. other women of the house, a daughter or personal slave attendant) to observe the hunchback on the reverse. For the secondary viewer, a curious play of visual imagery ensued: the image of the hunchback replaces the image of the primary be-holder, or coexists in the same field of view. A viewer is thus presented with two extremes of appearance: the beauty of the be-holder and the unsightly deformed hunchback. A viewer might thereupon situate herself somewhere along this sliding scale, or, read differently, having the ugly hunchback in direct opposition to the beauty of the be-holder would make any homely viewer feel pretty in comparison. Thus, part of the appeal of this mirror and its figural decoration arises from the viewer's recognition of the ease with which beauty and ugliness could slide unsteadily into one another (indeed, it serves as a reminder that beauty eventually fades). This mirror draws out tensions in looking, much in the same way as the hunchback now in the Villa Albani-Torlonia (cat. no. **32**), with his handsome face and deformed body, or the hunchback now in the Museum für Kunst und Gewerbe in Hamburg (cat. no. **33**), with his deformed but precious (bronze with silver inlay) body; these representations force a viewer to reconsider the meaning of the body of the hunchback and the function of his representation.

The evidence examined thus far clearly points to one reason why an individual might want to own a representation of a hunchback, whether that be statuette, mosaic pavement or bronze mirror: as a charm to protect their premises and themselves against the evil eye of envy. But it has also shown that these representations, while serving an apotropaic function, could take on additional meaning. Examining other representations in the corpus reveals a particularly charged reading, hitherto underexplored in contemporary scholarship on hyperphallicism: the hyperphallic Other as an object of sexual desire and titillation.

The erotic appeal of the hunchback

Although some scholars have argued that images of the hyperphallic Other were neither sexually stimulating nor seen as objects of sexual desire or titillation, evidence for the hunchback suggests that these images were stimulating to look at, and this stimulation could indeed play out erotically.[28] The erotic appeal of the (phenomenally) large penis is attested in a number of ancient, especially Latin, sources, though these stories are used chiefly as indicators of the perversion, and therefore Otherness, of those who seek out individuals so endowed for erotic titillation or sexual fulfilment.[29] Literature such as this is presumably stimulated by, and adds an extra layer to, the use of the hyperphallic Other as an apotropaion. We will therefore examine two examples of hunchbacks in the corpus, in association with extant literary evidence, to nuance the apotropaic reading of the hyperphallic hunchback.

A misbehaving hunchback

The most explicit example of the hunchback's association with an erotic context comes from a wall painting (cat. no. **16**) discovered in Pompeii.[30] This painting belongs to a large corpus of Nilotic scenes (over 130 in total), preserved on wall paintings and mosaic pavements, depicting dwarfs and pygmies, popularly used to decorate houses, baths, latrines and tombs in Pompeii, after the third quarter of the first century BCE.[31] This Nilotic scene depicts three male pygmies on a boat. The pygmy on the left is a hunchback, depicted standing and facing the two other pygmies. The hunchbacked pygmy wears a band around his head, similar to that worn by the hunchbacks in the British Museum in London (cat. no. **12**) and the Phoenix Gallery of Art in Geneva (cat. no. **14**), carries two (rhythm) sticks, of the same type carried by the hunchback (cat. no. **17**) and dwarf in the Antioch mosaics, and is ithyphallic.[32] Next to him is a pygmy bent on all fours with his buttocks in the air – he is in the coitus *a tergo* position – and looks as though he will soon be engaged in fellatio. Both he and the hunchback stare directly at the external viewer. The third pygmy reclines, head propped by his left arm, directly behind (literally, behind the buttocks of) the second pygmy; he smirks, and his gaze tells us why: it is directed straight ahead, at the buttocks of the pygmy, rather than turned towards the viewer. The scene is one of misbehaving pygmies, an orgiastic threesome on a boat sailing along the exotic, fertile Nile, fecund with fish and river flora. In the repertoire of Nilotic paintings, scenes of pygmies involved in sexual acts were particularly popular as decorations in the garden areas of Pompeian houses; the *a tergo* position was exclusive to scenes of lovemaking on boats, and is usually, though not exclusively, reserved for male–male encounters.[33]

The role of pygmies in such Nilotic scenes has been systematically studied by Clarke, Dasen and Versluys; all of whom agree that, in both a domestic and funerary context – that is in houses and tombs, especially in Italy where the greatest number of Nilotic scenes have been preserved – the representation of hyperphallic pygmies is to be attributed an apotropaic function.[34] For the average (male, citizen of a certain age, wealth and status) viewer these images of the hyperphallic Other (male, non-citizen and foreigner) engaged in sexual acts were meant to amuse and titillate; indeed, this contributed to their apotropaic power. As Clarke notes: 'By having them carry out sexual acts in open nature, artists created a comic foil to the elegant couples on beds who represented "bourgeois" lovemaking. The viewer of the Hellenistic period could identify him- or herself with the refined representations, but the expected response to the crude pygmies' acts would be laughter' (Clarke 1998: 43–4). According to Versluys, however, these images also had additional, erotic power. Versluys has suggested that scenes of sexual intercourse associated with the Nile flood referred to the importance of the Nile in Egyptian religion (namely the divine union between Isis and Osiris) and emphasized the pygmies' symbolism with fertility and abundance; rather than depicting comic parodies of lovemaking scenes, these were genuine imitations of foreign sexual-religious rituals (Mayboom and Versluys 2005: 182–202). Of course, the very foreignness of these individuals and their rituals could have been amusing to the Roman, i.e. Pompeian, audience, but here, too, the point is that laughter was not the only response that these overtly sexual images could elicit.

In this particular wall painting something more is going on. None of the pygmies are actually engaged in sexual activity, *yet*. The painting presents a moment (the so-called 'pregnant moment') at which the action stops and all three pygmies debate what to do next: the external viewer is thus implicated in this debate – confirmed by the two pygmies who stare directly at the external viewer – and is permitted to play out a range of possible outcomes. As a homoerotic scene, this underscores a male viewer's own erotic desirability, both to other men and to women. Given the importance placed on the role of active and passive sexual partners in the ancient world, this scene creates a tension by blurring the boundaries between soon-to-be-active pygmies and passive, but perhaps also soon-to-be-active, viewer. The context in which this wall painting was displayed (the triclinium? the peristyle portico?) and the events surrounding its viewing (e.g. a banquet or drinking party, perhaps with lavish entertainment, performed by deformed slaves? – see the previous chapter, and below) would certainly have affected a viewer's response to the scene. The sexual acts of the misbehaving pygmies thus make a deliberate statement about in/appropriate sexual conduct. However, in as much as this painting encourages the external viewer to take up a specific role or position (with one of the pygmies?) it also, by virtue of its two-dimensionality, ensures that the viewer remains at a safe distance from the events taking place – thus maintaining the role of an outsider looking in and affirming the difference between Self and Other.

A masturbating hunchback

The hunchback now in the Museum für Kunst und Gewerbe in Hamburg (cat. no. **33**) is remarkable in many ways, not least because of its overtly sexual and erotic nature. As we saw in the previous chapter, the decoration and detailing of this hunchback make him one of the finest in the corpus: this very small statuette, only 6.6 centimetres in height, is made of bronze, but both the eyes and the teeth are inlayed with silver. He is naked and emaciated, depicted seated on the ground with his legs spread symmetrically and crossed at the ankles.[35] His head is tilted downward and he appears with a sullen and dismal expression. Notably, he grasps the glans of his very large phallus with his left hand, masturbating.

The fact that this hunchback might at any moment ejaculate adds to his apotropaic power. It also emphasizes a very powerful auto-sexual act, which we cannot explain away as simply or solely apotropaic. An episode from the *Life of Aesop* is here informative, providing tantalizing evidence for the erotic appeal of the hyperphallic hunchback. In one scene of the *Life*, Aesop is caught masturbating outside his master Xanthus's house. Xanthus's wife stumbles upon Aesop and the sight of his penis, specifically its 'size and thickness', arouses her lust – so much so that she takes him as her temporary lover, demanding sex ten times:

> *Ἐν μιᾷ οὖν τῶν ἡμερῶν μονωθείς, ἐκδυσάμενος καὶ τὰς χεῖρας ἑαυτοῦ κροτῶν καὶ τινάσσων, ἤρξατο ποιεῖν τὸ ποιμενικὸν καὶ ἄτακτον σχῆμα. ἡ δὲ τοῦ Ξάνθου γυνή, ἐκ τοῦ οἴκου αἴφνης καταλαβοῦσα, φησίν 'Αἴσωπε, τί τοῦτο;' ὁ δὲ λέγει 'κυρία, εὐεργετοῦμαι καὶ τὴν γαστέρα ὠφελεῖ.' θεασαμένη δὲ ἐκείνη τὸ μῆκος καὶ τὸ πάχος τῆς αἰδοῦς αὐτοῦ, ἑάλω, καὶ ἐπιλαθομένη τῆς ἀμορφίας αὐτοῦ εἰς ἔρωτα ἐτρώθη.*

> One day when he was left alone, he stripped off and rattled and shook himself with his hands and began to act in a shepherdly and disorderly manner. The wife of Xanthus suddenly came out of the house and said, 'Aesop, what is this?', and he says, 'Mistress, I'm doing good work and it helps the womb'. And when this woman saw the size and thickness of his shameful parts, she was conquered and, forgetting his unshapeliness, was wounded with respect to love.[36]

We recall that the ugly and deformed Aesop was purchased as a *βάσκανιον* to protect his master's slave-shop from the evil eye of envy – nowhere in that episode, nor in other physical descriptions of Aesop in the *Life*, is the size of his penis mentioned as relative to his potency as an apotropaion (perhaps it was assumed a reader would simply know this). The importance of his penis lies not in its apotropaic agency, but rather, in that it is what makes Aesop sexually desirable to Xanthus's wife. The hyperphallicism, and indeed, hypersexuality, of this 'unshapely' hunchback slave leads to an illicit affair with a prominent and wealthy woman; moreover, it is through his sexual service, at least in part, that Aesop is able to earn his freedom.

Other literary evidence, too, indicates that the hunchback, even when not explicitly referenced as hyperphallic, seems to have been the target of sexual conquest. To the story of Aesop we can add the episode recounted by Pliny, and already mentioned in the previous chapter, in which a prominent and wealthy Roman woman, Gegania, falls in love with her hunchback slave, Clesippus:

> *Accessio candelabri talis fuit Theonis iussu praeconis Clesippus fullo gibber et praeterea et alio foedus aspectu, emente id Gegania eadem ostentante in convivio empta ludibrii causa nudatus atque impudentia libidinis receptus in torum, mox in testamentum praedives numinum vice illud candelabrum coluit et hanc Corinthiis fabulam adiecit, vindicates tamen moribus nobili sepulchro, per quod aeterna supra terras Geganiae dedecoris memoria duraret . . .*

> At the sale of a chandelier of this sort by the instructions of the auctioneer (named Theon) selling it there was thrown in as part of the bargain the fuller Clesippus a hunchback and also of a hideous appearance in other respects besides, the lot being bought by a woman named Gegania for 50,000 sesterces. This woman gave a party to show off her purchases, and for the mockery of the guests the man appeared with no clothes on; his mistress

> conceiving an outrageous passion for him admitted him to her bed and later gave him a place in her will. Thus becoming excessively rich he worshipped the lampstand in question as a divinity and so caused this story to be attached to Corinthian lampstands in general, though the claims of morality were vindicated by his erecting a noble tombstone to perpetuate throughout the living world for all time the memory of Gegania's shame.[37]

Although Pliny does not state the source of Gegania's *libidinis*, the fact that Clesippus appears naked certainly suggests that it *might* be the sight of his penis. Regardless of the cause, Gegania is harshly stigmatized because of her attraction to the hunchback, for Clesippus is no ordinary hunchback. Not only is he of a foul appearance, he is also a fuller. Gegania's desire for such a polluted creature adds to her *impudentia* and thus serves to highlight her own Otherness. This is very different from the stigma Xanthus's wife receives; Aesop, at least, is exceptionally clever and his overwhelming wisdom is appreciated by many. Clesippus, on the other hand, is appreciated by no one except Gegania. Such a place did this hunchback hold in Gegania's life that when she died, she left him her entire fortune!

Remarkably, Pliny's story is not the only record that survives about Clesippus: we have an inscription from that monumental tomb dedicated by the freedman Clesippus. A limestone *titulus* on the wall of a modern building on the Via Appia near Tarracina bears an epitaph with the name Clesippus Geganius along with his religious offices and civil service.[38] This tomb, while intended to commemorate Clesippus's new status, serves at the same time to highlight the stigma of his servile past and forever shames his mistress.

Although it is almost certain that any slave could have been obligated to submit to his/her owner's sexual demands, it seems to have been a common witticism in Latin literature to charge wealthy Roman women with being particularly demanding of sex from deformed male slaves; these women are thus stigmatized because of their (perverse) sexual proclivities.[39] Such stories cast women who lust after (deformed and hypersexual) men as non-normative, and they are to be understood by (male) readers as transgressive.

The stories of Aesop and Clesippus therefore add meaning to the masturbating hunchback in Hamburg, and indeed all representations of the hyperphallic hunchback; perhaps it warned a male viewer of the possible sexual appeal of the hunchback slave. If this were indeed the case, then the hunchback now in the Wurttemberg State Museum in Stuttgart (cat. no. **37**) might be thus contextualized: this bronze statuette, measuring 6.3 centimetres in height, depicts a nude hunchback sitting with his legs crossed, holding a string or leather thong to infibulate his large penis. Although the purpose of infibulation has been debated, its use in the Roman period to control sexual impulses, and as a means of contraception for slaves, could relate specifically to this hunchback.[40]

One final note must be added to the reading of the masturbating hunchback in Hamburg: in the previous chapter we explored the tactile appreciation of the hunchback in miniature and noticed a tension between looking and touching; this is played out most provocatively in this statuette. Getting 'caught in the act' adds friction to the tactile relationship between viewer and object; could the hunchback be taunting the viewer to both rub his hump *and* rub his penis? Based on the literary sources, we might suppose that such an invitation would be taken up by a female viewer of such predilection, adding another layer of meaning to the hyperphallic hunchback. All of this therefore puts the representation of the hunchback, both in the visual and literary records, within a larger cultural context of sexuality and eroticism.

The erotic appeal of the hunchback was not restricted to just slaves and those with low social status; but things seem to be rather different with the body of a bona fide citizen. In the *Lives of the Caesars*, Suetonius tells us that the emperor Galba's father, also named Galba, was both short of stature and hunchbacked.[41] Despite his physical appearance, however, he was an accomplished man: he had attained the consulship and was a rather famous litigator of the time. We will examine Galba more closely in the next chapter, but for our purposes here it is significant to note Suetonius's description of Galba's early encounters with his second wife, Livia Ocellina:

> *Uxores habuit . . .; item Liviam Ocellinam ditem admodum et pulchram, a qua tamen nobilitatis causa appetitus ultro existimatur et aliquanto enixius, postquam subinde instanti vitium corporis secreto posita veste detexit, ne quasi ignaram fallere videretur.*
>
> He married . . . later Livia Ocellina, a very rich and beautiful woman, who however is thought to have sought marriage with him because of his high rank, and the more eagerly when, in response to her frequent advances, he took off his robe in private and showed her his (deformed) body, so as not to seem to deceive her by concealing it.[42]

The exposure of Galba's hump is, if we believe Suetonius, at least one source of Livia's lust for Galba. Livia is to some degree stigmatized for this; Suetonius does not say as much, but presumably he would not have had to, because his readers would have been familiar with a wider tradition of other, more famous and scandalous, stories about women and hunchbacks (as above). Moreover, the fact that Livia's cognomina is Ocellina, 'small-eyed', may indicate that she suffered from a visual handicap, further contributing to her own stigmatization and characterization as Other. This episode may also shed further light on the story recounted by Pliny: perhaps it was not the sight of Clesippus's penis that aroused Gegania's lust, but rather his hump. Thus, the invitation to rub the hunchback's hump may have resonated sexually for certain viewers.

All of these examples, in art and literature, demonstrate that in considering the use of grotesques as apotropaia, the hunchback in particular complicates any such straightforward reading: while it fulfils an apotropaic role, there is also compelling evidence for other complementary functions; some were, to be sure, sexually stimulating and titillating. Classifying the hunchback as merely an apotropaion explains away his deformity, together with all other features. When we consider the context and *look* at the gesture and posture of the hunchback as well as the addition of other attributes, alongside the phallus, then we are forced, as the ancients must also have been, to re-evaluate the place of the hunchback in Hellenistic and Roman society.

4

Men who are not Men: Gendering the Hunchback

A disproportionately high number of representations of the hunchback are male in gender: of the fifty-five representations catalogued, all but two are male. Indeed, males are represented in greater numbers across all subsets of ancient representations of Other, especially of the deformed and disabled type, and most noticeably in representations of the hunchback, suggesting a deliberate motive behind this (male) gendered representation. Why, and how exactly, was gender important to the representation of the Other, and the hunchback in particular?

This chapter examines the construction of gender in ancient art by deploying detailed analysis of the male and the female hunchback. We examine, first, representations of the male hunchback, evaluating the masculinity of this marginalized male body, attempting to reconstruct the experience of what it was like to inhabit such a body. Examining both visual and literary evidence we will demonstrate that these representations reflect cultural attitudes about male identity and desirability in the Hellenistic and Roman worlds. We then move on to examine the two representations of female hunchbacks, analysing their iconography within the wider gamut of female abnormality, specifically with relation to images of obesity and old age. Contextualizing these images in terms of their ancient viewership, we will demonstrate that these female hunchbacks emphasize a sliding scale of beauty and ugliness, demanding a viewer question the aesthetic appeal of, and (erotic) response to, the female body. Moreover, this chapter places representations of the hunchback in the wider socio-cultural environment in which they were viewed to think about the place of the real-life hunchback in Hellenistic and Roman antiquity.

The male Other: the male hunchback

As Foxhall commented in 1998, 'the history of classical antiquity is a history of men' (Foxhall and Salmon 1998: 1). Likewise, the history of ancient art has been largely a history of the (idealized, beautiful and able) male body: traditionally it is the male body that has been privileged as the locus for reconstructing ancient identity.[1] Thus for Osborne, Kroisos, the Archaic kouros from the Anavysos cemetery in Athens, is fundamental in thinking about death (Osborne and Goldhill 1994; Osborne 1998a: 75–80, 1998b: 23–42); for Stewart, the ideal youths on the Parthenon frieze are central to understanding Athenian politics (A. F. Stewart 1990, 1997); for Bartman, the 'sexy boys' of Roman sculpture are critical for understanding Roman sexuality (Bartman 2002); and for Zanker, images of the emperor, especially Augustus, are key to unlocking imperial politics, power and propaganda (Zanker 1998, 2010). Certainly over the last few decades the emphasis has shifted from male to female bodies; indeed, there have emerged numerous cultural histories of the body that have been examined through the lens of gender and women's studies.[2] Nevertheless, open any contemporary introductory textbook or survey of Greek and Roman art and it is the faces (and bodies) of men with which you will be confronted.[3] Given the patriarchy of the ancient (and, indeed, modern) world, this is hardly surprising.

This book, too, has focused on the male body, but its aim has been to stretch our understanding of that body into territory less familiar: the deformed and disabled male Other. It is clear from looking at the corpus of hunchbacks that the extant evidence itself favours the male body over the female body, but unlike most (idealized) representations of the male body, the hunchback in a social, political and even religious sense is different: these males are not men who matter. With few exceptions, they depict the bodies of non-citizens: slaves, foreigners and the socially marginalized, who frequently performed the role of entertainers, or who have, for whatever reason, succumbed to begging. Thus, these hunchbacks are marginalized not only by their physical deformity (and other physical features), but, moreover, by their behaviour. They represent the antithesis of the restrained, self-controlled, beautiful male, the *kalos kagathos* or *vir bonus*, of Greco-Roman antiquity.[4] Their marginalization thus contributes to the ways in which they were viewed and the meanings derived from that viewing.

The possession of an identifiably male body was what privileged men – legally, politically, socially, etc. – above women in the ancient world. As Montserrat notes, 'A man's physical characteristics were explained in terms of his innate male claim to physical superiority . . . But it is important to remember that in the ancient world, not all men possessed the same category of the body' (Montserrat 1998: 153). What connects all of the male hunchbacks catalogued is that they are ugly in appearance; that is, they are all marked by somatic difference from the ideal Greco-Roman body type. This is manifest in a number of ways. The most obvious is the hunchback's physical deformity; but it is not just his hump, for he is often deformed in other respects too, dwarfed in corporeal proportion or exhibiting (caricatured) black African features. Other features also serve to exaggerate the hunchback's Other status: he has distorted facial and bodily features, pitiful expressions revealing a sullen mood or pain and suffering, bodies contorted in awkward positions, both standing and seated, either with arms or legs flailing in the midst of a dance movement, or burdened by objects carried. Most often these men are nude, or wear garments indicative of their non-citizen status: a loincloth or a tunic. This lack of appropriate clothing also emphasizes the male hunchback's second most outstanding physical feature: he is more often than not endowed with a large phallus, which either hangs flaccid or points erect.

Thus, across the corpus generally, we observe that in spite of the obvious gender of these hunchbacks, their masculinity is negated through their establishment as Other via their non-ideal physical characteristics – even their penises, the most obvious physical hallmark of masculinity, are distorted so as to deny their human masculinity in favour of something more animalistic – and their non-normative poses and gestures. As we shall see, through the use of four examples (cat. nos **8**, **9**, **25** and **34**), the male hunchback's representation hinges on his (mostly lowly) social status and thus contributes to our understanding of the function and meaning of the (representational and real-life) hunchback in Hellenistic and Roman antiquity.

The hunchback beggar

The hunchback now in the Antikensammlung in Berlin (cat. no. **34**) represents the lowest social class of the hunchback: the hunchback as beggar. This small, bronze statuette of a seated hunchback measures 16 centimetres in height – large in comparison to the majority of hunchbacks because of the rocky base upon which he sits, measuring 9 centimetres. Of unknown provenance and dating to the third century BCE, the hunchback is bald and his naked body is emaciated, with thin, atrophied limbs. His hump is ridged with the nodes of the spine clearly articulated, looking like a dorsal 'fin'. The hunchback is also represented as ithyphallic, though his penis is now partially missing.

This hunchback, one of the few in the corpus that has received attention because of its distinct appearance, has been analysed from a 'scientific' and 'social' perspective. The first perspective adopts a medical approach, analysing the hunchback's anatomy and deformities: Stevenson (1975: 234, 245) and Grmek and Gourevitch (1998: 217–18) argue that he suffers from Pott's disease. The second perspective adopts an art-historical approach, analysing the hunchback's pose and gesture: Masséglia argues that the frail body of this crippled hunchback serves less as an indicator of a pathological condition and more as an indicator of social status, in this case, the hunchback's lack of status (Masséglia, *Body Language*, Chapter 4).

The hunchback's seated pose and the position of his arms is characteristic of that used for slaves and beggars; given his nudity, it is likely that this is a poor beggar, since slave bodies are frequently adorned with some form of clothing.[5] The fact that this hunchback is seated on a rock further underlines his liminal status: sitting on the ground is part of a complex classification of gestures that aim at total self-abasement.[6] His facial expression adds to this: it is one of suffering, intended to evoke pathos, particularly if this hunchback does indeed represent a man ill with Pott's disease. Zanker, in his seminal book *Modes of Viewing in Hellenistic Art and Poetry*, has shown that suffering and the presentation of physical pain was exploited in sculpture of the Hellenistic period and this was done to manipulate a viewer's intellectual and emotional responses (Zanker 2004: 152, 167).[7]

Given the diverse range of body types depicted in the Hellenistic period, and the emphasis on realism, this hunchback may reflect the reality of the diversity and poverty of the city streets of Hellenistic (and Roman) city centres; indeed, ancient sources paint a picture of these multicultural cities where an assortment of diverse types of people lived, differentiated by skin colour, body type, language and so on.[8] Although we do not have a secure archaeological provenance for this piece, the subject matter of the hunchback beggar nevertheless reflects Hellenistic tendencies of representing ordinary men (and women) and 'the man on the street', thus reinforcing hierarchies of social status and reminding a male viewer of his own privileged status, good fortune and good health.

Thus, this hunchback beggar, who may have been used as an apotropaion, and touched by its viewers, is a male, but not a man; a male gendered beggar whose socially constructed gender is decidedly not male, unlike 'normal'-bodied males with social status.

The hunchback slave

The hunchback in the Museum of Antiquities in Toulouse (cat. no. **25**) also depicts a hunchback of low status: the hunchback as slave. This small, bronze statuette of a standing hunchback measures 6.9 centimetres in height, is of unknown provenance, and dates to the late Hellenistic to early Roman period. The hunchback is bald, has a short-cropped beard and lip moustache, and wears a loincloth around his waist that does little to conceal his large penis. He carries a cockerel in his right arm, which appears to be pecking at his chin, and a *lagynos* in his left hand.

This hunchback belongs to a small group of similarly represented figures in the corpus (see cat. nos **21–6** and likely **50** too), all of which carry the cockerel and a *lagynos*, a type which is found across many representations of Others in addition to hunchbacks. These figures have traditionally been interpreted as votives to the god Asclepius, possibly as dedications for improved health, or as charms to boost sexual potency, on the basis that the hunchback carries a sacrificial animal, the cockerel, and a libation, which would have been offered to the god; problematically, however, none of these representations have been found in votive contexts.[9] Others have interpreted these statuettes as representations of the hunchback's participation in the *lagynophoria*, a Dionysian festival introduced by Ptolemy IV Philopator at the end of the third century BCE in Alexandria.[10] The festival was popular among the lower social classes and even included slaves. Participants were expected to bring their own wine and food; thus the representation of the cockerel, the sacrificial animal of the poor, and the *lagynos*, the wine-jug, carried by the hunchback. Wrede interprets the figure of the crippled *lagynophoros* as the expression of the comical sphere of the Dionysian realm (Wrede 1991: 167f.), and Laubscher believes that such representations were intended to convey an arrogant attitude towards the lowest social strata and their involvement in religious cult (Laubscher 1982: 76ff.). If these interpretations are correct, then this hunchback also reinforces hierarchies of social status by means of religious differentiation. He too is a male, but not a man; a male slave whose religious practices ran decidedly opposite to the normal-bodied males of citizen status.

The hunchback entertainer

The hunchback now in the Metropolitan Museum of Art in New York (cat. no. **8**) also highlights the humble status of the hunchback, but reads rather differently. This small, bronze statuette of a standing hunchback, measuring 10 centimetres in height, is said to have been found on the Esquiline hill in Rome and dates broadly to the first century BCE–CE. The hunchback wears a short tunic, through which both hump and penis are clearly indicated, and thong sandals. His hair is elaborately rendered, formed by sheets of foil, made of copper alloy with an admixture of silver, laid in sections over the surface with curved incisions used to indicate the short strands of hair. The whites of his eyes and his two protruding teeth are silver and the little buttons on the sleeves of his tunic are made of the same copper–silver alloy as the hair.

This statuette was first analysed and published by Richter in 1913, who identified it as a mimic actor (Richter 1913: 154).[11] For Richter, the excellent execution of this statuette transformed it from an ugly and deformed figure into a work of high art. Indeed, the high quality of workmanship and the use of precious metals suggests that this was an object of art worthy of display. If the statuette does indeed depict a character of the mime, or perhaps, better still, the Dossenus of Atellan farce popular during the Roman period, then perhaps it functioned as a souvenir. As a souvenir, the statuette would continue to evoke memories of the vulgarity and buffoonery of the mime or farce, and bestow ongoing festive hilarity. At the same time, however, it is certain that an ancient viewer would have recognized the (negative) stereotypes associated with ancient actors: their profession marked these men as dishonourable or *infames* ('lacking in reputation'), even those who may have held Roman citizenship.[12] Thus, while serving as a source of amusement and entertainment, this statuette also reminded a male viewer of his own privileged social status and wealth; this is affirmed by the cost afforded to such a 'lowly' subject.

The hunchback citizen (?)

Things are slightly more complicated with the hunchback now in the Walters Art Gallery in Baltimore (cat. no. **9**); the social status of this hunchback is more difficult to determine. This small, bronze statuette of a standing hunchback measures 8.9 centimetres in height, is of unknown provenance – but thought to come from Cairo – and dates to the Hellenistic period. This hunchback, like the hunchback in New York (cat. no. **8**), is also remarkably detailed in his representation but has none of the same caricatured facial (or bodily) features and is not hyperphallic. Bald except for wavy locks above the ears, he is, if not handsome, at least not as ugly as the examples thus far examined. His furrowed brows suggest that he is in thoughtful contemplation; the pupils of the eyes, indicated by circular cuttings, highlight his gaze: he stares directly at the viewer. His clothing too is different from any other representation in the corpus: he wears a belted tunic, the hanging folds of which are clearly defined and through which we can clearly see his hump. Likewise, even his pose is unique. He raises his right arm above his head; his left arm is bent at the elbow with forearm raised and hand clutching an indeterminate object. He appears in the pose of a public speaker, or some other professional occupation with associated social status.

That this hunchback may indeed represent a public figure of status suggests a more complex reading of the representation of the hunchback; one that is augmented by extant literary sources. In Suetonius's *Life of Galba*, we are told that the emperor's father was both short of stature and hunchbacked. He is also described as having attained the consulship, and although only an indifferent speaker, was an industrious pleader at the bar.[13] This same Galba is mentioned twice by Macrobius in his *Saturnalia* in the context of the courtroom. These references reveal that Galba, although a man of status and generally good reputation, was nevertheless the object of derision because of his physical deformity, the hump on his back.

In the first instance from Macrobius, we hear the following:

> *Galbae, cuius informe gibbo erat corpus, agenti apud se causam et frequenter dicenti: 'Corrige, in me si quid reprehendis,' respondit: 'Ego te monere possum, corrigere non possum.'*
>
> To an ugly hunchback named Galba, who was pleading in court before him and kept saying: 'If you have any fault to find, correct me,' he [Augustus Caesar] said: 'I can offer you advice, but I certainly can't correct you.'[14]

In the second instance:

> *In Galbam, eloquentia clarum, sed quem habitus, ut supra dixi, corporis destruebat, M. Lollii vox circumferebatur: 'Ingenium Galbae male habitat.'*
>
> *In eumdem Galbam Orbilius grammaticus acerbius inrisit. Prodierat Orbilius in reum testis. Quem Galba ut confunderet, dissimulata professione eius, interrogavit: 'Quid artium facis?' Respondit: 'In sole gibbos soleo fricare.'*
>
> A jest that went the rounds was one directed by Marcus Lollius at the distinguished speaker Galba, who (as I have already remarked) was hampered by a bodily deformity: 'Galba's intellectual ability is ill-housed.'
>
> The same Galba was the victim of a crueller sheer from Orbilius the schoolmaster, when the latter came into court to give evidence against a defendant. Galba, seeking to disconcert the witness, pretended to be unaware of his profession and asked him: 'What is your job?' The reply was: 'Currying hunchbacks in the sun.'[15]

The same Orbilius, who himself seems to have been somewhat of an anomaly in that he lived to be nearly a hundred, is also said to have used a similar line against another well-known hunchback of the day, Varro Murena, a Roman general and politician of the first century BCE.[16] According to Suetonius:

> *Ac ne principum quidem virorum insectatione abstinuit; siquidem ignotus adhuc cum iudicio frequenti testimonium diceret, interrogatus a Varrone diversae partis advocato, quidnam ageret et quo artificio uteretur, gibberosos se de sole in umbram transferre respondit; quod Murena gibber erat.*
>
> He did not even refrain from gibes at men of distinction; for when he was still obscure and was giving testimony in a crowded courtroom, being asked by Varro, the advocate on the other side, what he did and what his profession was, he replied: 'I remove hunchbacks from the sun into the shade.' Now Murena was hunchbacked.[17]

The context for these remarks remains obscure, but both are jibes at the physical deformity of Galba and Murena, highlighting the humour exploited by the 'normal'-bodied towards men even of high social status. In such a context, we may read some representations of the hunchback, and specifically the hunchback in the Walters Art Gallery in Baltimore, as a representation of a man with status, but a man who is still unlike the normal-bodied male citizen and is thus marginalized because of his non-normative appearance. The examples of Galba and Murena provide additional significance when considering the reception of hunchback representations: ancient viewers would have had knowledge (either first- or second-hand) of actual hunchbacks living in their own communities and society, and certainly brought to bear the associations with those real-life hunchbacks when viewing these representations.

The hunchback: representation and real life

The examples discussed demonstrate the variety with which the male hunchback was represented and prompts us to question how a male viewer of the hunchback would have made certain observations about social status, wealth and health. Given that masculinity was an integral part of Hellenistic and Roman social status, ascribing that privileged gender to hunchbacks would have in turn ascribed a certain degree of status to them as well, without some machinations to negate that gender. Thus, ancient artists used the iconography of lower social statuses like beggars, slaves and entertainers, exaggerated non-ideal physical attributes, and hyperphallicism to distance the biological masculinity of the hunchback from the socially constructed, privileged masculine ideals of its viewers. Indeed, even in the case of a hunchback with real social status, as exampled by Galba and Murena, the deformed male is marginalized with verbal barbs in order to distance him from a normal, privileged, masculine gender.

This is the realm of representation. How, if at all, does the representation of the hunchback reflect what it may have been like to actually live with a physical deformity, a prominent and visible hump on one's back, in the ancient Hellenistic and Roman worlds? And how did 'normal'-bodied people understand and relate to hunchbacked people? Examining other evidence, particularly skeletal remains and mortuary practices, in association with current disability studies theory, may shed further light on attitudes towards the real-life hunchback.

Graham (2013) has recently demonstrated that what was considered a 'normal' body in the ancient Roman world was very different from our traditional understanding; indeed, 'disparate', or deformed and disabled bodies may have been much more visible in the general population, and thus less a spectacle than their characterization in representation might imply (see also Rose 2003). Skeletal remains survive from across the Roman Empire – in Italy, from the suburbia of Rome, and at Herculaneum, as well as the Roman provinces – revealing that crooked bodies were likely more common than straight ones. The ancient Romans not only suffered from disfiguring congenital and infectious diseases that caused significant spinal deformities, such as tuberculous spondylitis, or Pott's disease, but other, less debilitating diseases, such as osteoporosis, which caused kyphosis or curvature of the spine.[18] It may be the case that hunchbacked individuals, of all types, i.e. those suffering from severe spinal disease, or 'merely' a hunched back on account of old age, were visible, and vital, members of the community, but their representation, for whatever reason, is skewed towards the grotesque in the visual record.

Rose has also demonstrated that disparate bodies in ancient Greece were much more visible in the general population, and moreover, that individuals with a wide range of disabilities could be equitably integrated into the community, rather than excluded.[19] The hunchback may have been a more active member of Hellenistic and Roman society; this can be attributed to the strong network of interdependence that extended beyond the family to the wider community.[20] Generally, a hunched back had little impact on one's ability to perform in most occupations; though without doubt, individuals who were severely hunchbacked may have been more restricted, depending on their status and wealth. A hunched back alone did not bar an individual from entry to prominent professions: Galba and Murena are evidence of this, although, admittedly, these men are of an elite class of citizens with more privilege than most. Hunchbacked individuals of the lower classes may have had fewer options available; these individuals could have found employment as entertainers, as documented in the corpus. Some of these hunchbacks may have become household pets, given the Roman penchant for owning slaves with unusual physical features and obvious physical deformities, as discussed in Chapter 2. It is also probable that a number of hunchbacks, especially those suffering from diseases that disabled them in other ways, would have faced unemployment and financial hardship, seeking charity by begging, also documented in the corpus.

Thus, when approaching representations of the (male) hunchback, ancient viewers were not simply presented with some kind of fantastic, alien and imaginary form with little or no antecedent in the real world. Instead, these representations were caricatures of people within their own communities. An unresolved and resonating tension is thereby created between the viewer and the hunchback: the Othering of hunchbacks through these representations would have, by extension, Othered real-life hunchbacks in the minds of the viewers. Conversely, any normalization of real-life hunchbacks would have been reflected back on the Othered represenations by viewers. So it would seem that the sliding scale between the deformed hunchback and body beautiful from the representational world plays out in the real world, too.

Othering the female hunchback

So what of the female hunchback? Only two representations of female hunchbacks survive (cat. nos **10** and **45**). By and large, representations of women displaying physical deformities in classical art are relatively few. Take, for example, representations of dwarfs. Although a significantly larger number of representations of dwarfs have survived than representations of hunchbacks, only a limited number of these depict females. Garmaise calculates a three-to-one ratio of male to female dwarf statuettes from the Hellenistic and Roman periods, and suggests that one reason why representations of male dwarfs are favoured over female dwarfs is because they possess the potential for, and frequent display of, phalluses (Garmaise, *Dwarfs*, 128–9). This implies that the primary motivation behind the production of representations of dwarfs was to serve as apotropaic talismans; while this was certainly one function, and perhaps the most common, it was not the sole function, as Garmaise himself recognizes. In her study of dwarfs from ancient Egypt and Greece, Dasen suggests that the absence of female dwarfs indicates that female malformation was felt unpleasant or disquieting and may also bear witness to some sympathetic feelings, since their representation would have implied making them objects of popular derision (Dasen, *Dwarfs*, 204). This, however, supposes that it was acceptable for male dwarfs to be objects of popular derision, but not female. Why would female deformity have been considered taboo? Or, why could the conventions of representation not admit female deformity to the same extent as male deformity?[21]

Despite the vast amount of research on (the role, status, and importance of) women in antiquity, no in-depth study has considered the representation of female abnormality and/or deformity and disability.[22] While such a study is beyond the scope of this book, the existence of two female hunchbacks in the corpus nevertheless demands explanation. It is therefore necessary to examine, albeit briefly, the meaning of female abnormality in antiquity so as to contextualize the two female hunchbacks in our corpus.

Only two of the hunchbacks here catalogued are represented as female. The first hunchback, now in the Louvre in Paris (cat. no. **10**), is depicted with her hands clasped at her chest. She wears an elaborate garment that is draped over and partially covering her head, which is crowned with an ivy wreath. Notably, she is one of a few representations of old age in the corpus. The second hunchback, also in the Louvre (cat. no. **45**), is depicted squatting on the ground holding a *kantharos* or drinking cup, usually for wine, in her hands and she too wears an ivy wreath. She is also the only representation of obesity in the corpus.

Evidence for female deformity and disability in antiquity is relatively meagre. In the literary sources, two brief passages from Herodotus's *Histories* provide the bulk of information on deformed and disabled women.[23] Both accounts occur within a 'foreign' context; however, they rely on the presumption that a Greek (and later Roman) audience would have understood their implications because of similar understandings of physical deformity. The first comprises an account of the Babylonian marriage market, in which ugly and deformed females are provided with a dowry by the profits of pretty females and publicly auctioned to men who cared little for beauty. The second comprises an account of a lame Bacchiad woman named Labda, who, although bound by intermarriage, is rejected by her kinsmen and betrothed to a certain Aetion, descendant of the Lapiths. Both accounts demonstrate that anomalous physical traits, such as ugliness or deformity, did not necessarily prevent a woman from fulfilling her two most important socially prescribed roles as wife and mother. Rather, they reveal that such physical traits were perceived as unsightly in a female and devalued her aesthetic, and actual, worth.

It is this aesthetic value that is perhaps the most obvious reason for the lack of representations of female deformity in the artistic record. We must remember that ancient society was one in which artistic production was predominantly controlled by men and oriented primarily towards the male viewer. Just as the male body depicted man, not as he actually was, but how he could or should be, so too did the female body misrepresent woman by idealizing her. That said, there do survive a number of representations depicting females with socially ascribed abnormalities, such as old age and obesity.[24] Unlike the more awful human afflictions of disease and deformity, old age and obesity seem to have been more acceptably represented. But how then are we to reconcile the two female hunchbacks in our corpus which are at once physically deformed *and* socially marginalized? We must examine these two hunchbacks within the wider gamut of representations featuring obesity and old age.

Representations of obese women seem to have been fairly popular in antiquity, especially in Hellenistic terracottas.[25] As the majority of these representations lack secure archaeological contexts, their function has been the source of continuous debate, with a variety of competing interpretations having been proposed. Traditionally they have been linked to fertility because of their pronounced sexual features, i.e. large breasts and wide hips, which are conducive to child bearing; however, a number of additional, more controversial, theories have also emerged.[26] Thompson argued that some of these figures might represent old hetairai, or courtesans, 'who entertained guests by dancing burlesques' (Thompson 1954: 91). Charbonneaux (1936: 20) has suggested that they were offerings deposited at healing sanctuaries by women who were eager to lose weight. Garland has even suggested that they reflect a taste for larger women on the part of Greek males.[27] These theories, however, in addition to lacking conclusive evidence, perhaps better reflect modern stereotypes or prejudices rather than ancient attitudes. What this evidence seems to demonstrate is that obesity in representations of women was not negatively perceived; the obese female hunchback was likely not necessarily an object of derision.

Representations of old women also seem to have been common from the Hellenistic period onwards.[28] Perhaps the most famous extant representation of female old age is the Drunken Old Woman in Munich.[29] The old woman is represented seated on the floor and clutching a *lagynos*, or wine-jug, decorated with ivy on its shoulder, thus placing it as a gift of Dionysos (Fantham 1994: 177–9; Biers 1996: 303).[30] The woman has a bony chest, sagging breasts and a wrinkled face.[31] She wears a tunic which appears to have slipped off her right shoulder, recalling the *Aphrodite Kallipygos* discussed in Chapter 1, perhaps, as Smith notes, serving as a mock-coquettish reference to her vanished sexual attraction (Smith 1991: 137–8), or, as Beard suggests, recalling Aphrodite herself, now long past her prime, and thus serving as 'a joke about beauty itself, and its desirability; a put-down for women, no doubt, but also a sneer at male desire' (Beard and Henderson 2001: 142). This seems to demonstrate that old age in representations of women was not *in itself* negatively perceived; here it is the fact that this old woman is drunk and cannot control her behaviour.

This comparative material highlights yet another aspect of the blurring and overlapping in iconography in the corpus of hunchbacks. Both of the female hunchbacks wear wreaths upon their heads and one figure squats clutching a *kantharos*, thus recalling the 'Drunken Old Woman'. This suggests that perhaps they too are to be associated with the Dionysian world, and thus re-enforces the idea, introduced with the hunchback *lagynophoros*, that the hunchback was somehow incorporated within the Dionysian cult. Based on all of this, therefore, we might argue that images of females exhibiting gross physical deformities were frowned upon, unless these had certain religious associations. Whatever their intended function, these representations of female deformity, old age and obesity presented a deliberate contrast to their youthful, idealized counterparts and underlined the interaction between beauty and ugliness which lay at the very heart of visual desire and aesthetic appeal. Moreover, it is certainly not coincidence that the two female hunchbacks in our corpus are represented as old and obese; because these female hunchbacks cannot be endowed with phalluses, artists needed some alternative means of Othering these women, thus subverting any social status afforded to 'normal' women.

The ugly hunchbacked women are very different from the ugly hunchbacked men in the corpus. While men reveal a wider range of ugliness, emphasized by caricatured facial features, distorted poses and grossly enlarged genitals, there are far less liberties in representation taken with the female hunchback. Of course we cannot make sweeping conclusions given the limited nature of the evidence, but it seems that one key aspect of their representation is the availability, or unavailability, of phalluses as marker of gender and thus status. Since the female hunchbacks do not have phalluses, they are already at a lower social status. However, to make sure they are sufficiently marginalized, the female hunchbacks are represented with at least one alternative Othering characteristic, taken from a pre-existing tradition so as to be recognizable to ancient viewers, thus obesity and old age. Likewise the representation of the male hunchback was also built on a pre-existing tradition of Othering, namely association with dwarfs and black Africans and lowly professions, like actors or entertainers.

Gender thus played a significant role in the reception of hunchback representations. Beyond the more obvious and exaggerated characteristics of the hunchback, gender was perhaps the most relatable aspect of their representation, due to the existing cultural and social framework and consequent gender-related status in ancient society. If indeed hunchbacks were more normalized and integrated into society, the negation of gender and associated status in these representations was perhaps critical to their function as good-luck talismans: Otherness was directly tied to apotropaic function. Without obscuring the normalization and humanization of gender, viewers were in danger of relating to, and perhaps even sympathizing with, the hunchback as a fellow community member.

Conclusion

This book has focused on *looking* – looking at the Other using representations of the hunchback as linchpin. So, what's in a hump?

In the category of deformed and disabled Other, the hunchback has, up until now, received relatively little scholarly attention, a significant omission in this burgeoning field of research. As we have seen, the wealth of surviving evidence for the hunchback in both the literary and visual records demands attention. By cataloguing representations of the hunchback, and including images and descriptions thereof, I have sought to make them widely and readily accessible for reference and study so that we can once again begin to see the hunchback as the ancients did. The catalogue serves as an intrinsic element of, and stimulus for, the case studies which have been analysed in this book, the implications of which reach far beyond the hunchback – beyond even the Other – and touch upon broader issues in the study of ancient art.

The hunchback is unique in the category of Other; his identity is immediately and unmistakeably recognizable because of the hump (whatever shape and size it may take) protruding from his back. The hunchback's hump is the (optic and haptic) point of focus in his representation, yet, as we have seen, one cannot look at his representation without recognizing the deliberate iconographic blurring with other Others: the hunchback often appears dwarfed in corporeal proportion or possesses certain black African characteristics. It seems that ancient artists relished blurring the boundaries between these different types to stress both difference *and* similarity, emphasizing the ease with which they could slide unsteadily into one another. The categories of normality and abnormality were continually shifting, forcing a viewer to constantly re-assess the division between Self and Other as it relates to their own body and that of the hunchback (or black African, or dwarf, etc.).

We see in all of these representations a fascination with that which is different – black skin colour, a dwarfed body, a humped back – and an emphasis on displaying these different bodies so as to highlight normative values associated with physical appearance and social status. These non-normative bodies were titillating to look at and indicate that there was a certain fascination with confronting the abnormal, whether that be to point at it or applaud it. This titillation and fascination still resonates today: the 13 November 2014 online issue of the *Daily Mail* featured an image of the world's tallest man, Sultan Kösen, measuring 8 feet, 1 inch tall, meeting, for the first time, the world's shortest man, Chandra Dangi, measuring 21.5 inches (Figure 13). Posing outside the Houses of Parliament in London to commemorate Guinness World Record Day, the duo shake hands and wave to the crowd who have come to see 'The VERY odd couple'.[1] Their handshake suggests a mutual acceptance and appreciation of Otherness, and their image, on display for us as viewers, encourages a similar acceptance and appreciation of their extraordinary corporeality. But more than this, this image and, indeed, these individuals also demand that a viewer question his or her own body type and somatic normality against these extremes; in this respect, we are not so far removed from the ancients.

Of course, images of the Other and the way in which they are viewed vary considerably across cultures and time. What, then, were the intentions and implications of representing such individuals in the ancient Hellenistic and Roman worlds? Given the paucity of archaeological evidence regarding the production and display of representations of the hunchback, it would be impossible to adopt any single comprehensive or conclusive explanation for their function and meaning; indeed, as demonstrated in the preceding chapters, representations of the hunchback were put to many different uses depending on the whims, inclinations or beliefs of those who owned and/or viewed them. Though particularly popular in the private sphere where they (in two and three dimensions) commonly decorated domestic spaces, the meaning of the hunchback was dependent on the eyes viewing and hands touching.

But despite the varied use of these representations, a common underlying motive behind the production, purchase and display of the hunchback seems to have been rooted in an ancient superstition that continues to endure today. In modern Italy and the wider Mediterranean, the lucky hunchback is a popular superstitious phenomenon; in ancient Roman culture, the hunchback

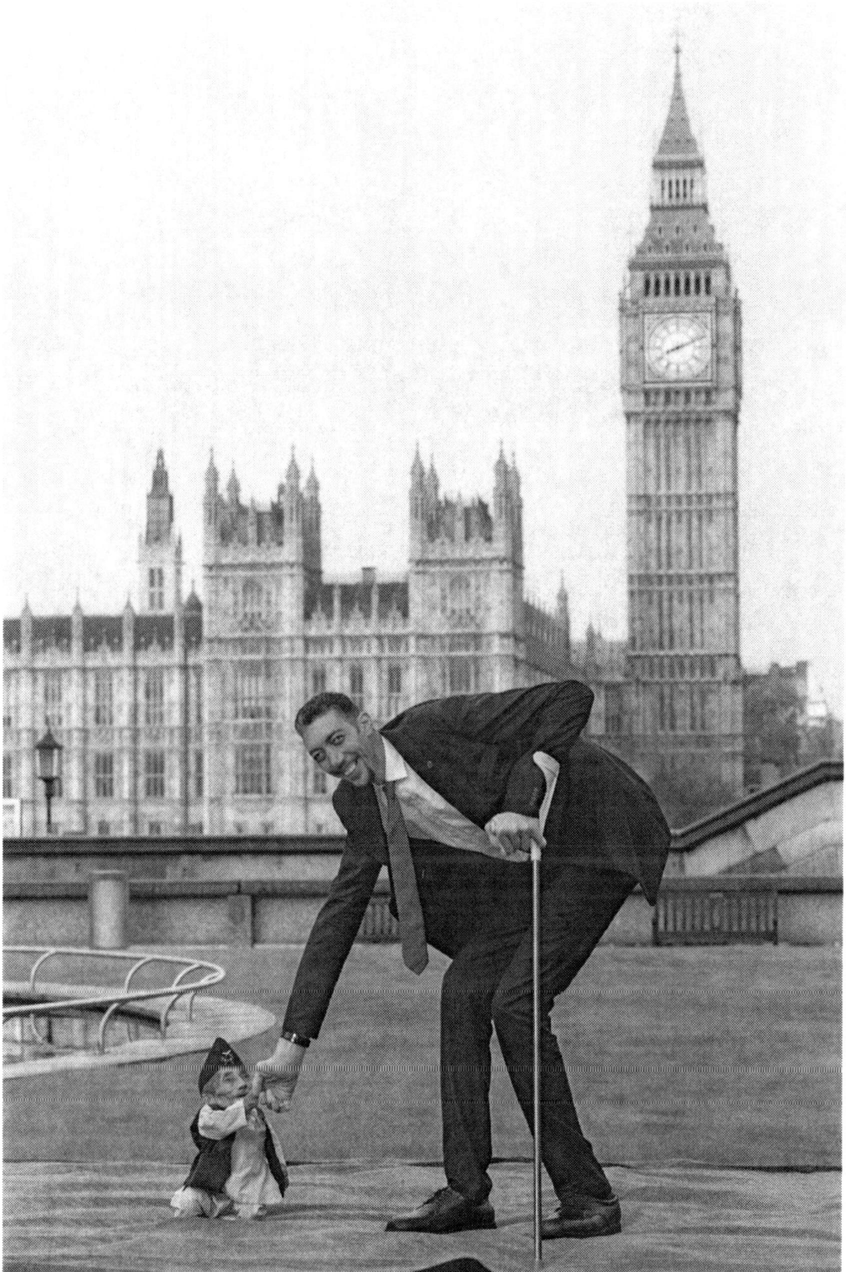

Figure 13 'The VERY odd couple': photograph from 13 November 2014 depicting the world's tallest man, Sultan Kösen, meeting the world's shortest man, Chandra Dangi, in London, UK.

was also considered lucky.[2] We have already seen that a great part of the appeal of these representations, particularly in sculpture, was the invitation to rub the hump of the hunchback, presumably for good luck, or some other (unknown) purpose. Literary evidence also teems and teases with the possibility of the lucky hunchback, suggesting that a hump was symbolic of good fortune. Perhaps the most compelling evidence for this comes from Suetonius. In his *Life of Domitian*, Suetonius informs readers that before Domitian's death he dreamt that a golden hump grew from his back and he regarded this as 'an infallible sign that the condition of the empire would be happier and more prosperous after his time'.[3] Indeed, as Suetonius recognizes, this was soon shown to be true through the stable and benevolent rule of the Nerva–Antonine Dynasty. It's clear that readers too would have understood the meaning of the growth of a golden hump – a lucky sign of future prosperity.

The hunchback is indeed lucky as represented in the corpus: in miniature sculpture, when touched and caressed, the hunchback elicited laughter and festive hilarity; in the mosaic pavement from Jekmejeh, the hunchback warded off evil; on the Etruscan mirror, the hunchback was taken from life into death, safeguarding its owner even in the afterlife. In all of these examples, the hunchback acted as an inverse symbol of the viewer's luck, affirming his privileged health, wealth and social status: everything that the *hunchback is not* serves as a stark and explicit validation of everything that the *viewer is*, or at least teases out the distance in between.

On the whole, then, a viewer's encounter with these hunchback representations was a resonant, and, in some ways, a reciprocal one: recognizing the Otherness in the hunchback necessitated a recognition of the Self in relation to that Otherness, whether in opposition *or* in alignment. By rendering the hunchback in a permanent medium, either as a miniature statuette, a large-scale sculpture or as decoration on a vase painting, wall painting, mosaic pavement or mirror, the hunchback was, in a sense, brought under control, allowing him a place among the 'normal'-bodied. The high quality of workmanship and decorative detail of the hunchback indicates a level of care and appreciation that, in some ways, legitimized his ugly appearance and lowly social status. As such, these representations elicited a variety of responses from their viewers, ranging from light-hearted amusement to thought-provoking moral introspection. Moreover, they functioned as stimuli to promote conversation among viewers – whether that be in the form of educated debate or uncouth banter – and contemplation – about the place of this deformed body, and all bodies, including a viewer's own, in contemporary society.

All of this demonstrates that representations of the hunchback are clearly good to think with and can greatly enhance our understanding of ancient art and culture: the hunchback was as much a signifier of the Other as it was of the Self; similarly, ancient culture can be understood as much through the deformed body as the body beautiful.

The Catalogue of Hunchbacks

Each entry in the catalogue has the following format: the first line provides the catalogue number, current museum or gallery location and corresponding accession number. When available, photographs are indicated by a star (★) next to the catalogue number and are to be found in the plates immediately following. All photographs are courtesy of the respective museum or gallery, unless otherwise indicated in the photo credits. Below this are biographical details: the preserved dimensions of the piece, given in centimetres and using the abbreviations H for height, and when available, W for width and D for depth, its date (if known), its provenance, which, when presented in *italics* should be regarded with caution, details of previous ownership, and the present condition of the piece including additional information regarding inlay or traces of paint. This is followed by a brief description of the piece and concludes with a short bibliography of relevant sources. The bibliographical references are intended to be informative rather than exhaustive. Sources which provide only a brief mention of a specific piece are not included, unless this is the principal reference. This format is a standard plan; minor variations occur in entries where information is neither available nor particularly extensive. Although every piece is treated individually, overlap does occur between representations that are closely related iconographically.

I. Hunchbacks standing and/or stooping

A. Hunchback, standing and/or stooping, nude

Bronze figurines

1. Cairo, Museum of Egyptian Antiquities, 27707.
H. 7.5cm – provenance unknown. Purchased February 1889.
Right arm, left hand and lower part of both legs missing.

Left hand raised; very thin limbs, large phallus, beardless and bald except for a side-knot.
Bissing, *AA* 1903: 149, fig. 4n; Edgar and Cowan 1903: pl. V.

2.★ Vienna, Kunsthistorisches Museum, VI, 169.
H. 8.0cm – 2nd century BCE – provenance unknown. Purchased in 1819.
Polished bronze with a black patina.
Left hand rests on advanced left leg, right hand clenched at thigh of right leg. Thin limbs, large phallus, bald, protruding chest box.
Wace 1903–4: 105, B7; Yeames 1907: 281, fig. 2; Nicoll 1931: 89, fig. 82.1.

3. Louvre, Paris, Br 708.
H. 7.5cm – provenance unknown. Davillier bequest, 1885.
Hands and feet partially missing.
Hands bound behind back. Dwarfed body, large phallus, large head (with caricatured features), bald but wavy locks above the ears and lower back of the head, bearded.

Terracotta figurines

4. Paris, Louvre. Originally Fouquet Collection, 456.
H. 9.6cm – from Memphis, Egypt.
Dwarfed limbs, double hump, protruding chest box.
Perdrizet 1921: 162, pl. 107.

5.★ Munich, Antikensammlungen, TC/SC 306.
H. 19.0cm – provenance unknown.
Feet missing, nose broken on left side. Hole in the hump used for suspension.
Standing with hands loosely clasped on chest. Large ears and caricatured facial features (nose, lips, eyes), long neck, emaciated body, ithyphallic and bald.
Sieveking 1930: 19, pl. 19, 1; Dunbabin and Dickie 1983: 20.

B. Hunchback, standing and/or stooping, semi-nude

Bronze figurine

6. Copenhagen, National Museum, ABa40fra.
H. 9.1cm – provenance unknown. Purchased from the Guldberg Collection, 1810.
Dark green/black patina.
Both arms, left leg below the thigh and right foot are missing.
Stooping hunchback wears a loincloth. Large phallus, bald, protruding chest box.
Wace 1903/4: 105, B1.

C. Hunchback, standing and/or stooping, draped

Bronze figurines

7. Cairo, Museum of Egyptian Antiquities, 27710.
H. 7.7cm – *from Egypt*.
Stooping hunchback wearing a tunic with a cloak.
Edgar 1903: no. 27710, pl. 5; Reinach 1920–30: IV, 355, no. 4.

8.★ New York, Metropolitan Museum of Art, 1912, 12.29.6.
H. 10.0cm – c. 50 BCE–50 CE – found on the Esquiline hill in Rome, 1727.
Both forearms missing. Crown of head inlaid with copper-alloy and silver admixture. Teeth silvered.
Wears a sleeved tunic with a fringed border and sandals. Hump and large phallus visible through garment. Large head, caricatured features (large ears, hooked nose, crooked mouth and whiskers), slightly protruding chest box.
Murray 1898: 164–7, no. 28; Richter 1913: 149–56, pl. 6.

9.★ Baltimore, Walters Art Gallery, 54.744.
H. 8.9cm – c. 332–32 BCE – *from Cairo*. Purchased before 1931.
Cast; vent hole on left thigh. Broken above knees and across the right wrist. May have been silvered. Pupils of eyes indicated by circular cuttings.

Wears a belted tunic and raises his right arm above his head; left arm is bent at the elbow with forearm upraised, fingers closed over an indeterminate object. Bald except for wavy locks above the ears.
Hill 1949: 72, no. 151; Eichler 1951: 61; Reeder 1988: 139, no. 54.

Terracotta figurine

10.★ Paris, Louvre. Originally Fouquet Collection, 458.
H. 14.6cm – from Smyrna.
Traces of red paint on body.
Old woman. Wears a long garment with a hood and a crown or wreath upon her head. Hump is clearly visible through the fabric of her drapery. Hands are clasped at chest.
Perdrizet 1921: 163, pl. 107.

D. Hunchback, dancing, nude

Bronze figurines

11.★ Toulouse, Museum of Antiquities (Saint-Raymond), 25635.
H. 9.9cm – provenance unknown.
Fingers on both hands are partially broken. Both feet are restored.
Stooping hunchback with a large phallus.
Reinach 1920–30: II, 563, no. 7; Grmek and Gourevitch 1987: 216, fig. 161.

12.★ London, British Museum. Payne Knight Collection, 1824.4–31.6.
H. 8.9cm – provenance unknown.
Lower legs, right arm and penis are missing. Eyes inlaid with gold and silver.
Left arm raised and bent with closed fist. Wears a tight fitted cap. Thin limbs, protruding chest box.
Wace 1903/4: 106, B23, fig. 2.

13.★ Geneva, Phoenix Gallery of Art, 17005.
H. 7.8cm – provenance unknown. Acquired in the early 1980s from the ex-Elie Boustros Collection.

Both hands are missing.
Bald, thin, elongated limbs, protruding chest box and a large phallus that points backward between the legs.
Reeder 1988: 141–3, figs 56–7; Vercoutter 1991: figs 297–8.

14.★ Geneva, Phoenix Gallery of Art, 20825.
H. 8.3cm – provenance unknown. Acquired on the German art market, 2007.
Arms and lower legs missing. Reddish brown surface of the bronze now covered by a green and black patina.
Wears a pointed cap held in place by a metal band decorated with a diadem, nude but wears a necklace around his neck, thin limbs and protruding chest box. Large phallus that points backward between his legs.
Aboutaam and Yubero 2007: 55.

15.★ Munich, Antikensammlungen, 4317.
H. 8.5cm – provenance unknown.
Both arms above the elbows and right foot are missing. Left handle of vase is broken.
Thin, elongated limbs, large phallus. Wears an upside-down vase on his head.
Lullies, *AA* 1962: 631, no. 17; Giuliani, *AA* 1987: 709.

Wall painting

16.★ Italy, Pompeii.
First century BCE from Pompeii. The painting no longer survives. Drawing has erect phallus of the hunchback expurgated.
Dwarfed hunchback standing on a boat with two other dwarf figures. Wears a band around his head and carries two rhythm sticks.
Carelli 1755–1831: 7: 297–9; Helbig 1868: 381, no. 1539; Kunz and Nippert 1986: 37.

E. Hunchback, dancing, semi-nude

Mosaic pavement

17.★ Antakya, Hatay Archaeology Museum, 1026a.
H. 0.84m × W. 0.83m – 2nd century CE – from the vestibule of a Roman villa at Jekmejeh.
Dwarfed hunchback with head turned looking over his right shoulder. Holds a rhythm stick in each hand, wears a loincloth and has an erect phallus.
Levi 1941: 220–32, pl. 56; Levi 1947.

F. Hunchback, playing an instrument, nude

Bronze figurines

18.★ Berlin, Staatliche Museum, Antikensammlung, 2142a.
H. 9.9cm – 1st century BCE – found at Cologne (Hahnentor area). Both feet missing.
Large phallus, bald, playing the flute or carrying rhythm sticks.
Wace 1903–4: 105, B2; Holländer 1912: 325, fig. 218.

19. Berlin, Antikensammlung Staatliche Museum, 2143.
H. 10.4cm – provenance unknown.
Both arms missing below the shoulders.
Similar to **18** above – also likely to have been playing the flute or carrying rhythm sticks.
Wace 1903–4: 105, B3; Holländer 1912: 325, fig. 217.

G. Hunchback, playing an instrument, semi-nude

Vase painting

20.★ Saint-Germain-en-Laye, National Archaeological Museum, 17888.
H. 21.0cm – 1st century CE – found at a Roman villa in the Rhône Valley, 1861. Purchased 1888 from M. Hoffmann.
Handle restored in the third century CE.

Body of vase depicts the scene of a feast in which one of the central characters is a hunchback flute-player wearing a short loincloth and a pointed cap.
Froehner 1873: 73, pl. 17–18 and 1886: no. 418; Goldman 1943: 22–34; Versluys 2002: 211–12, no. 110.

H. Hunchback, carrying a cockerel and/or a vase, nude

Bronze figurines

21. Louvre, Paris. Originally Gaudin Collection.
H. 7.5cm – 2nd–1st century BCE – *from Egypt.*
Carries a cockerel in right arm and a *lagynos* in the left hand. Bald except for back-knot, large phallus.
Charbonneaux 1962: 127, fig. 28.

22.★ London, British Museum, 1922.7–12.6
H. 7.5cm – from Egypt. Purchased at the Fouquet Sale, 1922.
Both feet and part of phallus are missing.
Carries a cockerel in right arm and a *lagynos* in the left hand; cockerel pecks at the hunchback's face. Wears a tight fitted cap, has a double beard and large phallus.
Perdrizet 1911: 59, no. 95, pl. 28.

23.★ Strasbourg, Archaeological Museum, 11.987.5.1
H. 7.0cm – 2nd–1st century BCE – from Rue du Vieux Marché aux Vins, Strasbourg. Purchased from J. J. Hatt, 1952.
Carries a cockerel in right arm and *alagynos* in the left hand. Cockerel pecks at the hunchback's face. Wears a tight fitted cap, has a double beard and large phallus.
Hatt 1954: 493, fig. 12; Picard 1958: 83–99.

24.★ Berlin, Antikensammlung Staatliche Museum, 8724.
H. 9.0cm – from Egypt. Former collection of Freiherr von Bissing.
Carries a cockerel in right arm and an unidentified object in the left hand (perhaps a castanet). Large phallus points backward between the legs. Wears an ivy wreath.
Wace 1903/4: 106, C4; Pernice, *AA* 1904: 38, fig. 15.

I. Hunchback, carrying a cockerel and/or a vase, semi-nude

Bronze figurines

25.★ Toulouse, Museum of Antiquities (Saint-Raymond), 25634 A.
H. 6.9cm – provenance unknown.
Right foot missing.
Carries a cockerel in right arm and a *lagynos* in the left hand; cockerel pecks at the hunchback's face. Bald and wears a loincloth around his waist.
Roschach 1865: no. 546; Grmek and Gourevitch 1998: 210, fig. 156.

26. Florence, Archaeological Museum, 2314.
H. 7.0cm – 3rd century BCE – from Alexandria.
Carries a cockerel with right arm and a *lagynos* in the left hand; cockerel pecks at the hunchback's face. Bald, large phallus and wears a loincloth around his waist.
Wace 1903/4: 106, B17; Grmek and Gourevitch 1998: 211, fig. 157.

J. Hunchback, carrying various objects, nude

Bronze figurines

27.★ Vienna, Kunsthistorisches Museum, VI,162.
H. 6.0cm – 2nd century BCE – provenance unknown. Purchased from Baron K. von Hess, 1808.
Right leg below knee and lower part of object in right hand are missing.
Left leg advanced forward, head looks over his right shoulder, body twisted towards the right. Left arm raised and bent at elbow, carries an unidentified object over his left shoulder and an unidentified object (bag?) in his right hand. Bald, large phallus.
Von Sacken 1871: pl. 46, 6; Reinach 1920–30: II, 566, no. 2.

28. Mainz, State Museum, AA8854.
H. 6.8cm – provenance unknown.
Stooping hunchback holding an unidentified object in extended right hand. Wears a cap and has a prominent scrotum.
Reinach 1920–30: V, 304, no. 3.

29. Lyon, Museum of Gallo-Roman Civilisation, A2002.
H. 7.0cm – provenance unknown.
Stooping hunchback carrying fruit in his right hand and an unidentified object in his left hand. Bearded, large phallus and large, hooked nose.
Reinach 1920–30: IV, 356, no. 2; Boucher 1970: 52, no. 30.

Terracotta figurine

30.★ Boston, Museum of Fine Arts, 01.7613
H. 10.4cm – late 3rd–2nd century BCE – *from Smyrna*. Purchased from E. P. Warren, 1901.
Traces of white slip on the body and red paint on the grapes.
Hunchbacked dwarf holding a bunch of grapes. Oversized head and brows, wide nose and mouth, thin, small arms.
Winter 1903: 447; Uhlenbrock 1990: 162; Garland 1995: fig. 47.

K. Hunchback, carrying various objects, draped

Bronze figurine

31. Amsterdam, Allard Pierson Museum, 7983.
H. 8.2cm – provenance unknown. Purchased from the Eddé and Scheurleer Collection, 1911.
Left foot missing. Right hand and left elbow are damaged. Rectangular piece of bronze crusted on the left thigh. Pupils and nostrils are hollow.
Stooping hunchback carrying a basket. Wears a chiton fastened over left shoulder and tucked below the thighs. Left arm is hidden under chiton. Bald except for a back-knot, ithyphallic.
Reinach 1920–30: V, 514, no. 2; Van Gulik 1940: 9, no. 15, pl. 30.

II. Hunchbacks seated and/or crouching

A. Hunchback, seated and/or crouching, nude

Marble sculpture

32.★ Rome, Villa Albani-Torlonia, 964.
H. 58.5cm (head 28.5cm) – 2nd century CE – from Baths of Caracalla in Rome, discovered in 1758.
Nose, right shoulder and back of the head are restorations. Left earlobe and left arm missing. Semi-erect phallus was removed and covered by a fig leaf.
Upper torso and head of a hunchback. Portrait-style head; he wears a long, trimmed beard with a lip moustache and has short, thick, curly hair, with a central part on the forehead. Semi-erect phallus, protruding chest box, stunted belly.
Bernoulli 1901: 54–6, pl. 7; Richter 1984: 78–80; Bol 1989: 227–31; Trentin 2009.

Bronze figurines

33.★ Hamburg, Museum für Kunst und Gewerbe, 1949.40.
H. 6.6cm – mid 3rd century BCE – provenance unknown.
Right arm and left foot missing; right leg and left arm bent out of place; crack in neck. Eyes and teeth inlaid with silver.
Seated with legs crossed holding his large phallus with his left hand. Bald head with top-knot, emaciated body.
Jantzen 1958: 47–51; Hoffman, *AA* 1960: 122, no. 35, figs. 54–56; Giuliani, *AA* 1987: 710–12.

34.★ Berlin, Antikensammlung Staatliche Museum, 30894.
H. 16.0cm – 3rd century BCE – *from Rome*. Former Castellani Collection.
Right foot, index finger and eye enclosure missing. Large phallus now missing.
Seated on a rock with legs crossed and hands clasped together. Bald head, emaciated body.

Neugebauer 1951: 69–71, no. 62, pl. 30; Jantzen 1958: 47–51; Giuliani, *AA* 1987: 702–5.

35.★ Hartford, Conn., Wadsworth Atheneum, 1917.817.
H. 8.3cm – 2nd century BCE – *from Alexandria*. Gift of J. Pierpont Morgan.
Seated on a rock with legs crossed in the style of a Spinario. Wears a *pilos* (cap), has thin limbs.
Reinach 1920–30: V, 537, no. 7; Keith-Bennet and Grierson 1980: 23.

36.★ Paris, Louvre, Br. 4382
H. 6.5cm – 2nd century BCE – from Egypt.
Seated with legs crossed in the style of a Spinario. Extremely emaciated but with well-defined musculature and a prominent pigeon breast.
Meige 1897: 815, no. 7; Reinach 1920–30: II, 816, no. 1.

37.★ Stuttgart, Württemberg State Museum, R 78,5.
H. 6.3cm – 1st century BCE – from a Roman villa in Herbrechtingen.
Young male sitting with legs crossed, holding string or leather thong to infibulate his large phallus. Large, bald head, thin limbs.
Hartmann, *AA* 1912: 13–16; Grimm 1969: 218, no. 133; Himmelmann 1983: 92, pls. 52/53.

Terracotta figurine

38. Paris, Louvre. Originally Gaudin Collection, CA 5190.
H. 7.5cm – from Smyrna. Gaudin gift, 1901.
Left arm broken at elbow, hand on right arm and both feet are missing. Holes for suspension on back. Traces of red paint on face and body.
Seated hunchback with pigeon breast, elongated limbs, large head (with caricatured features), ivy crown, very large phallus.
Besques 1971–2: 171, D1183, pl. 236a; Mitchell 2013: 285, fig. 10.

39. Paris, Louvre. Originally Gaudin Collection.
H. 6.6cm – provenance unknown.
Seated hunchback with pigeon breast. Bald head, emaciated body.
Winter 1903: 444, no. 5.

Ivory figurine

40.★ London, British Museum. Townley Collection, 1814.7–4.277.
H. 10.3cm – 1st century BCE – from Egypt.
Right hand missing. Figure carved separately from the base.
Seated on a pedestal with legs crossed and left hand resting on the knee. Head is large and sunken into the shoulders. Thin limbs, protruding chest box, close-cropped hair, large ears, corrugated forehead.
Barnett 1982: 65, pl. 66c; Yeames 1907: 279–82.

Bronze mirror

41.★ Tarquinia, National Museum.
H. 14.1cm × W. 13.8cm – 1st century BCE – from Etruria.
Seated hunchback with a bird perched on his extended right hand. Two birds appear perched above and to the right of the hunchback's head facing one another. Has a protruding chest box, erect phallus and feet are stumped (lame?). Surrounded by a circular pattern of double flora along edge of mirror.
Tabanelli 1963: 72, pl. 33; Gerhard 1995: V 186, pl. 141.1; Grmek and Gourevitch 1998: 217, fig. 162.

B. Hunchback, seated and/or crouching, semi-nude

Bronze figurine

42. London, British Museum. Payne Knight Collection, 1666.
H. 5.1cm – provenance unknown.
Sits in foetal position huddled on a triangular base raised on three legs. Wears a loincloth coiled around the waist and has a large phallus.
Wace 1903–4: 106, B22.

C. Hunchback, seated and/or crouching, draped

Terracotta figurine

43. Berlin, Antikensammlung Staatliche Museum, 8819.
H. 7.0cm – provenance unknown.
Left arm extended and wearing a himation, beardless, large phallus.
Pernice, *AA* 1904: col. 38.

D. Hunchback, carrying various objects, nude

Bronze figurine

44.★ Berlin, Antikensammlung Staatliche Museum, 8756.
H. 7.0cm – from Egypt. Gift of Freiherr von Bissing.
Wears a wide-brimmed hat and carries a bag over his left shoulder.
Wace 1903–4: 105, B4; Pernice, *AA* 1904: col. 38, fig. 14; Holländer 1912: 326, fig. 219.

Terracotta figurines

45.★ Paris, Louvre. Originally Gaudin Collection.
H. 8.5cm – from Kition, Cyprus.
Old, obese woman crouched in foetal position, holding a *kantharos* in her hands.
Richter 1902: 177; Winter 1903: II, 458, no. 3, Heuzey 1923: 192, pl. 10, fig. 3.

46.★ San Francisco, de Young Memorial Museum, 55106.
H. 15.2cm × W. 8.9cm – 3rd century BCE – provenance unknown.
Gift of M. H. de Young Endowment Fund.
Hunchback dwarf riding a donkey or goat and carrying fruit. Barrel shaped body, angular hump, oversized head and thin limbs. Bald head with full brows, nose and mouth.
Holländer 1912: fig. 220; Uhlenbrock 1990: 162.

47. Athens, National Archaeological Museum. Originally Misthos Collection.
H. 14.0cm – provenance unknown.
Hunchback dwarf riding a donkey or goat, carrying an unidentified object. Barrel-shaped body, angular hump, oversized head and thin limbs. Bald head with full brows, nose and mouth.
Holländer 1912: fig. 221; Winter 1903: 447, B9; Uhlenbrock 1990: 162.

III. Fragments of hunchbacks

A. Hunchback busts, in the form of hanging vases

Bronze figurine

48.★ Paris, Louvre. Originally Fouquet Collection, 96.
H. 7.9cm – from Egypt.
Bald but wears a wreath. Ears are pierced with holes indicating a suspension chain.
Perdrizet 1911: 59, pl. 28.

Terracotta figurine

49. Paris, Louvre. Originally Fouquet Collection, 459.
H. 9.0cm – from Alexandria.
Bald except for a top-knot. Attachment on top of head for a suspension chain.
Perdrizet 1921: 163, pl. 107.

B. Hunchback busts or torsos

Bronze figurine

50.★ Toulouse, Museum of Antiquities (Saint-Raymond), 25634.
H. 5.3cm – provenance unknown.

Both arms below the shoulders and legs below the knees are missing.
The figure likely carried a cockerel and vase, as his pose is similar to cat. nos 21–6.
Bald, wears a loincloth around his waist, ithyphallic.
Roschach 1865: no. 546; Grmek and Gourevitch 1998: 210, fig. 156.

Terracotta figurines

51. Paris, Louvre. Originally Fouquet Collection, 457.
H. 8.0cm – from Egypt.
Torso and head of a nude hunchback. Bald with large ears and a beak-nose.
Perdrizet 1921: 162–3, pl. 107.

52.★ Boston, Museum of Fine Arts, 01.7622.
H. 8.4cm – 2nd century BCE–2nd century CE – *from Smyrna.*
Purchased from E. P. Warren, December 1901.
Arms and legs missing. Traces of white slip and dark red on the body colour.
Head and torso of a hunchback. Protruding chest box, individualized head.
Perdrizet 1921: 162–3, pl. 107.

53. Paris, Louvre. Originally Gaudin Collection, CA 5640.
H. 6.7cm – from Smyrna. Purchased 1903.
Bust of a hunchback.
Besques 1971–2: 170, D1177, pl. 235a.

54. Paris, Louvre. Originally Gaudin Collection, CA 5642.
H. 8.0cm – from Smyrna.
Torso of nude hunchback with pigeon breast.
Winter 1903: 444, no. 8; Besques 1971–2: 173, D1216, pl. 242c.

55.★ Athens, National Archaeological Museum. Misthos Collection, 5558.
H. 8.5cm – from Smyrna.
Arms and legs missing.
Dwarfed hunchback. Bald head, protruding chest box.
Winter 1903: 444, no. 7.

Cat. no. 2

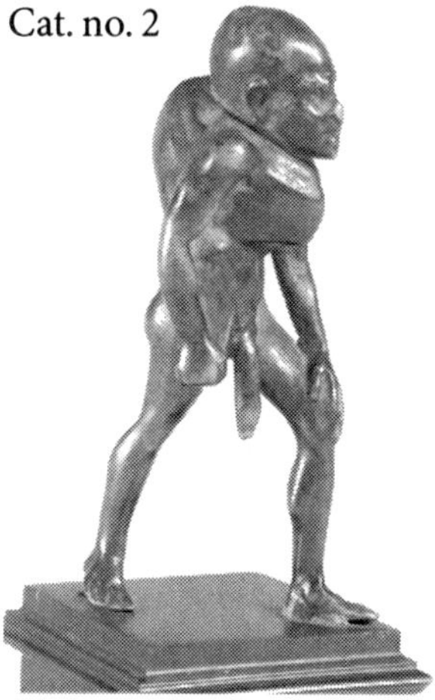

Cat. no. 5

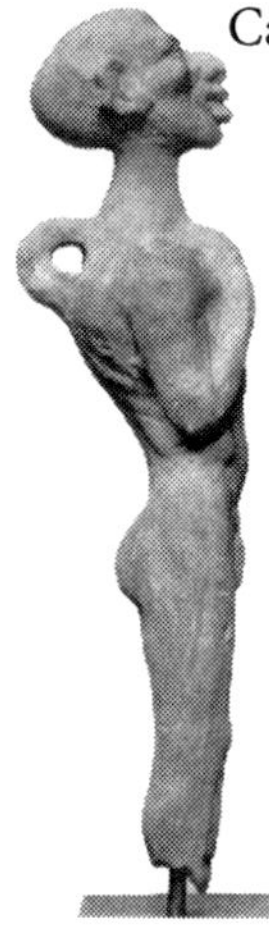

Cat. no. 8(1)

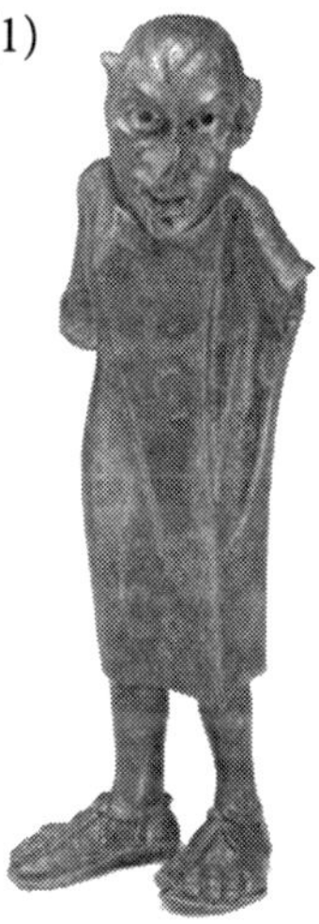

Cat. no. 8(2)

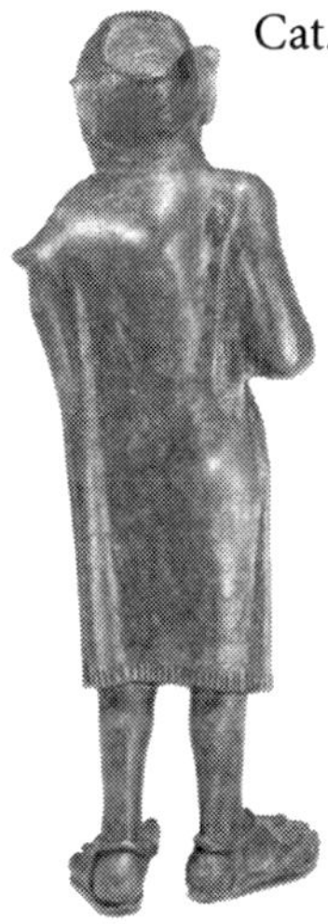

Cat. no. 9(1)

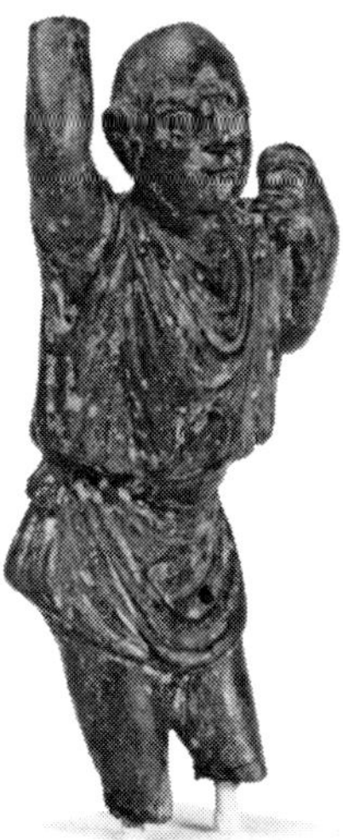

Cat. no. 9(2)

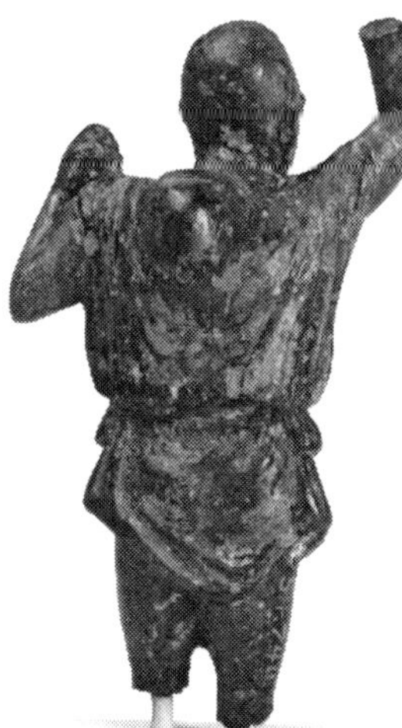

Cat. no. 10(1)

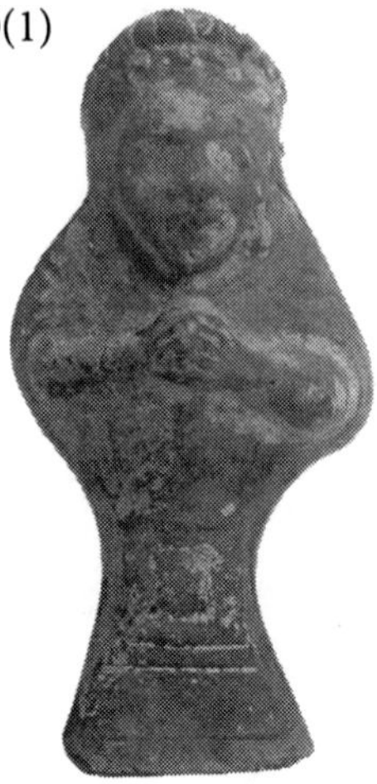

Cat. no. 10(2)

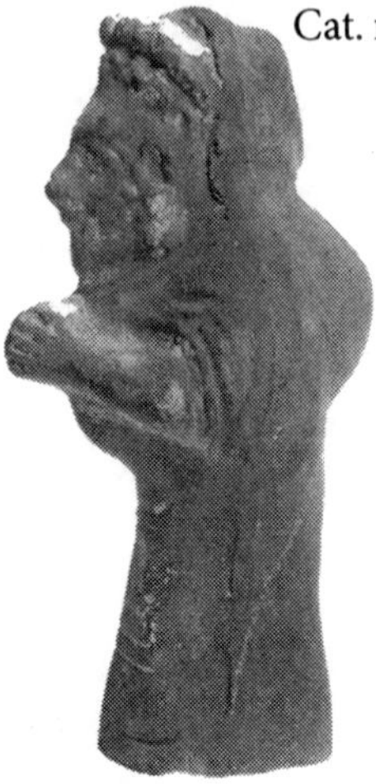

Cat. no. 11(1)

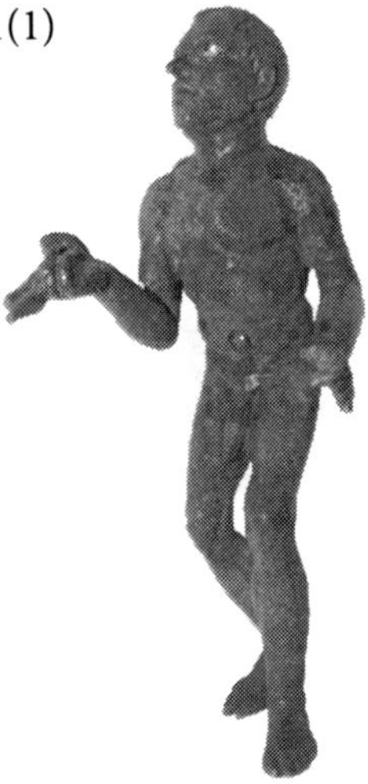

Cat. no. 11(2)

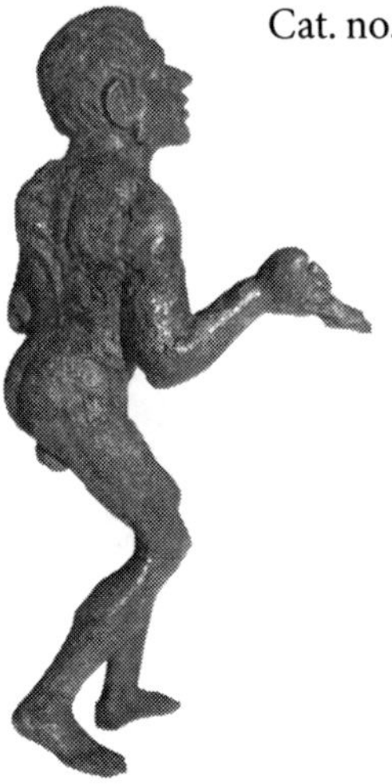

Cat. no. 12(1)

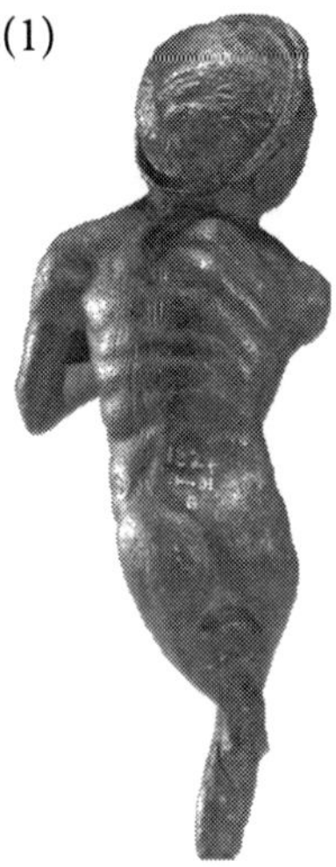

Cat. no. 12(2)

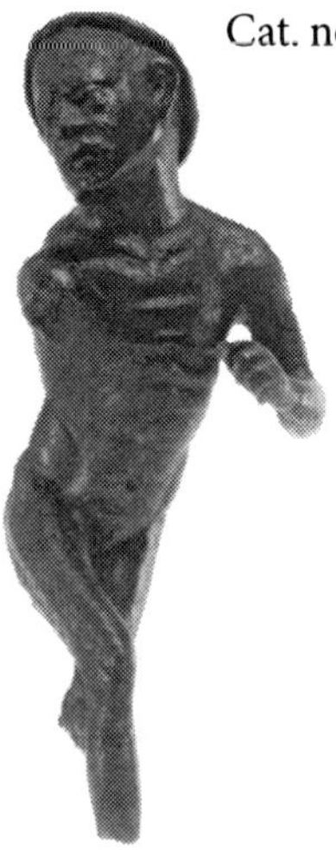

Cat. no. 13

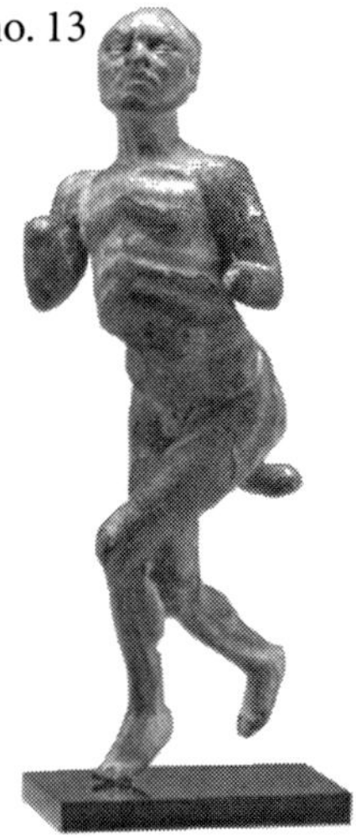

Cat. no. 14

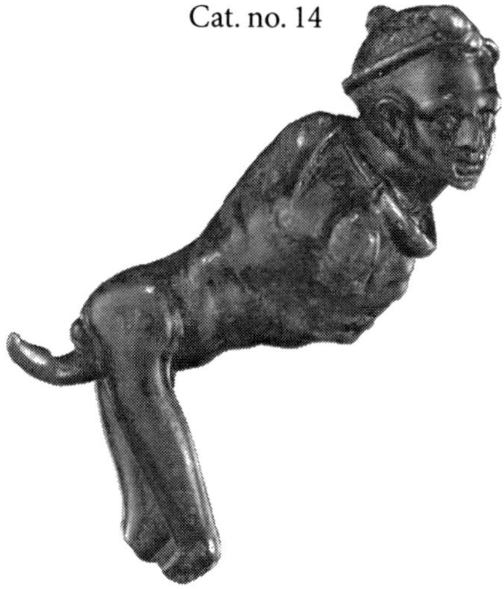

Cat. no. 15(1)

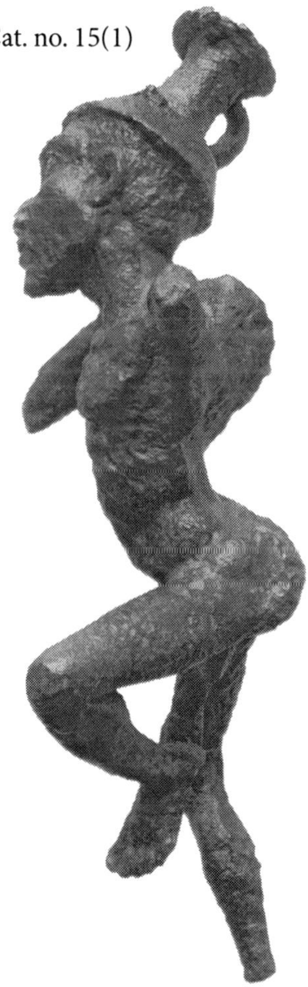

Cat. no. 15(2)

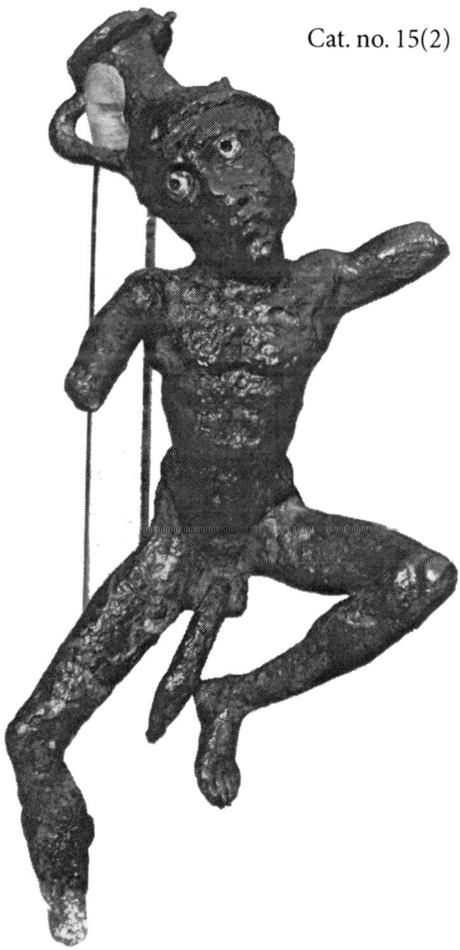

Cat. no. 16

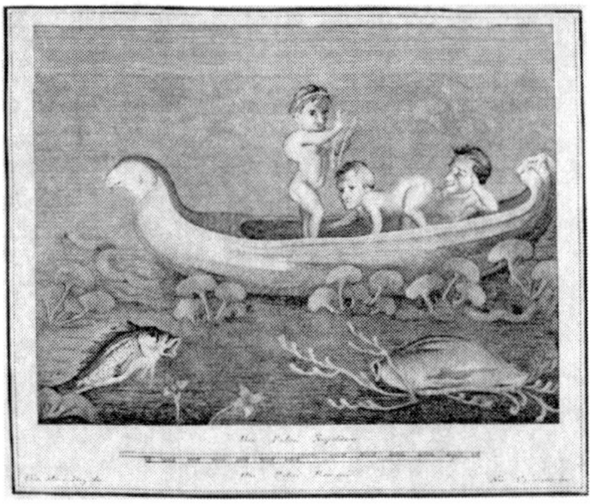

Cat. no. 17

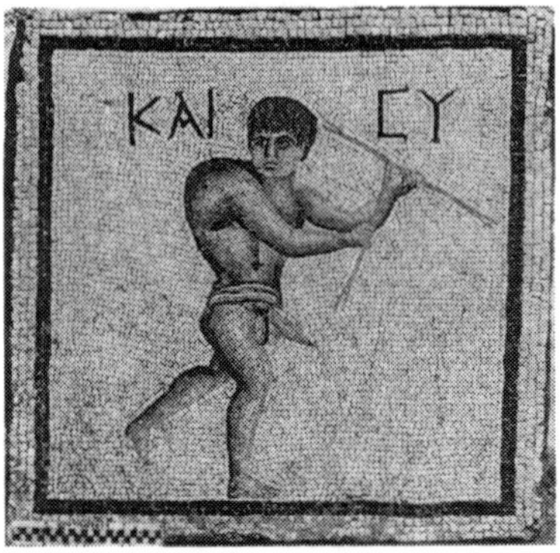

Cat. no. 18

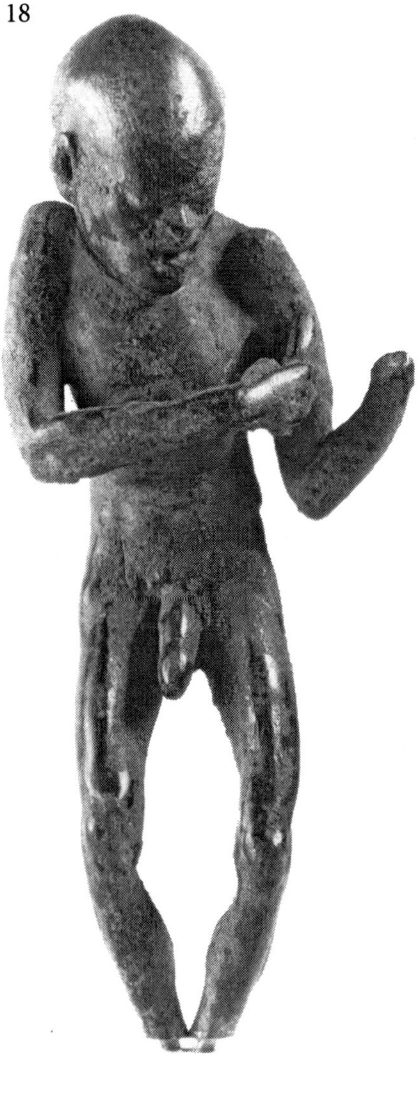

Cat. no. 20(1)

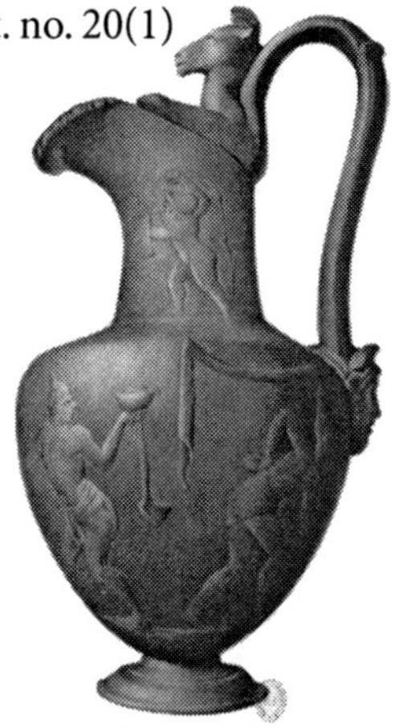

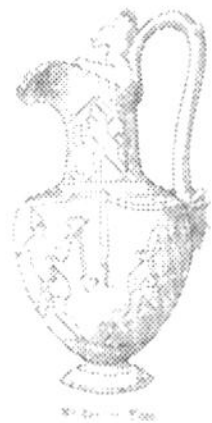

Cat. no. 20(2)

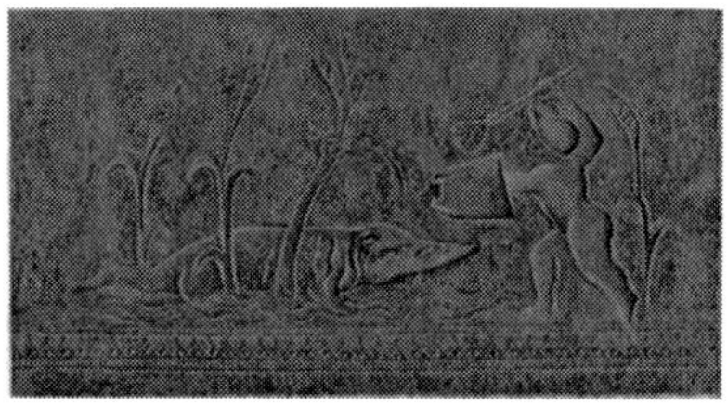

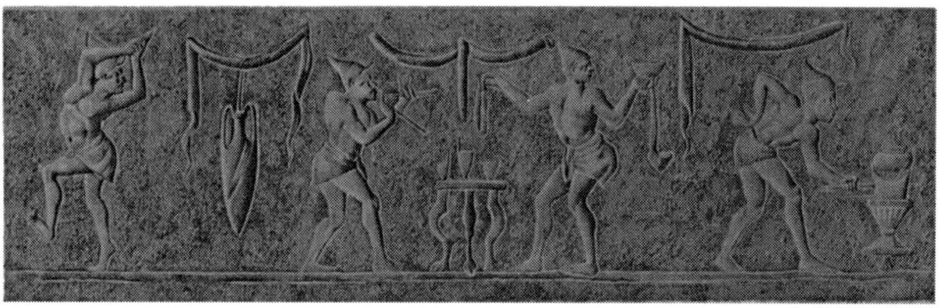

Cat. no. 22

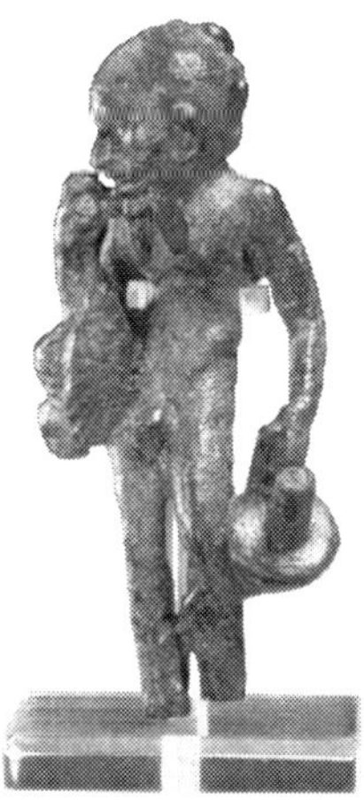

Cat. no. 23

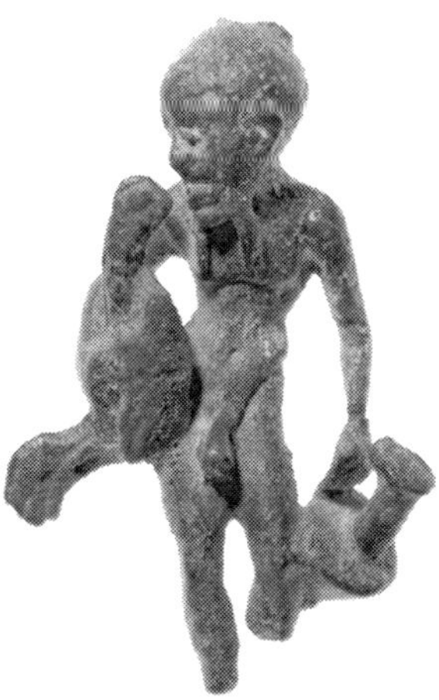

Cat. no. 24

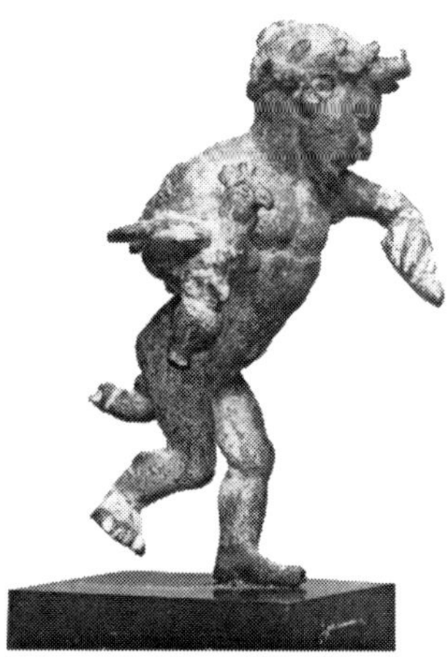

Cat. no. 25(1)

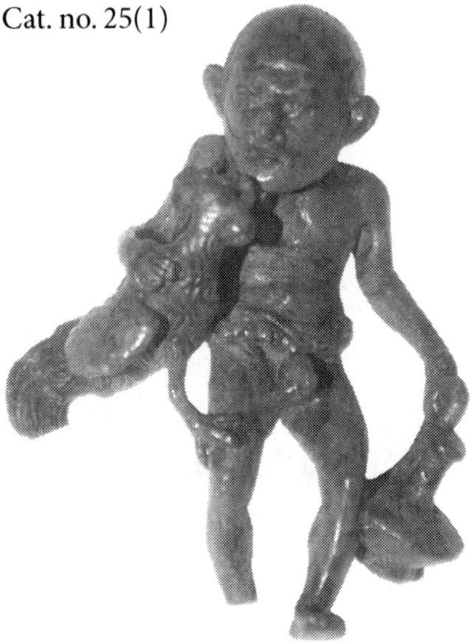

Cat. no. 25(2)

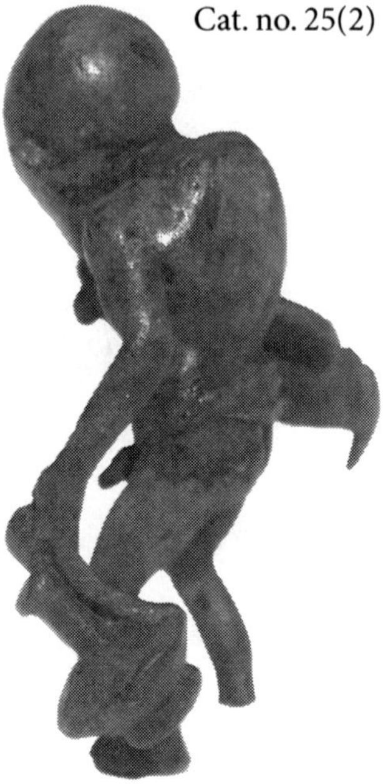

Cat. no. 27

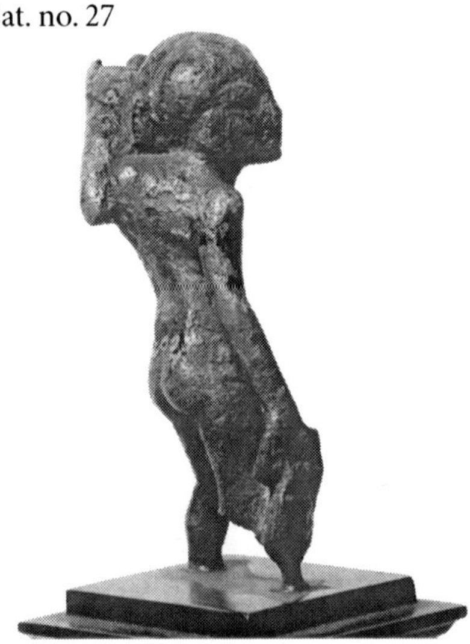

Cat. no. 30

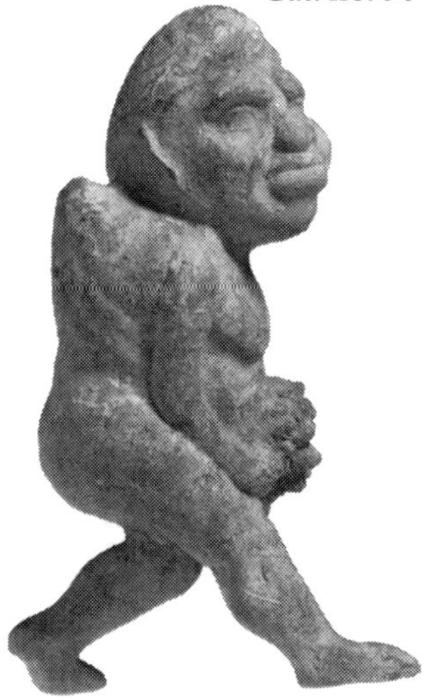

Cat. no. 32(1)

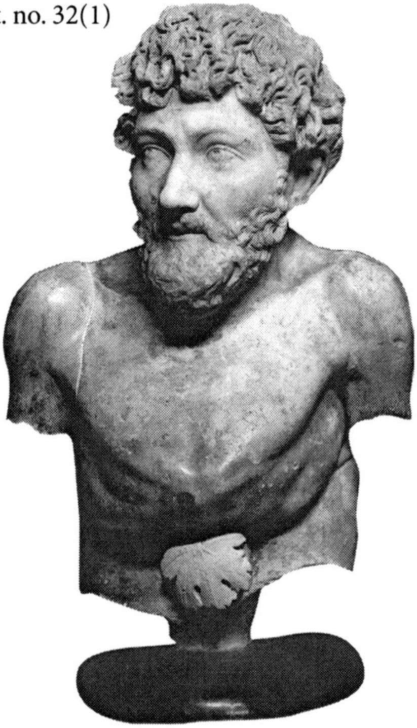

Cat. no. 32(2)

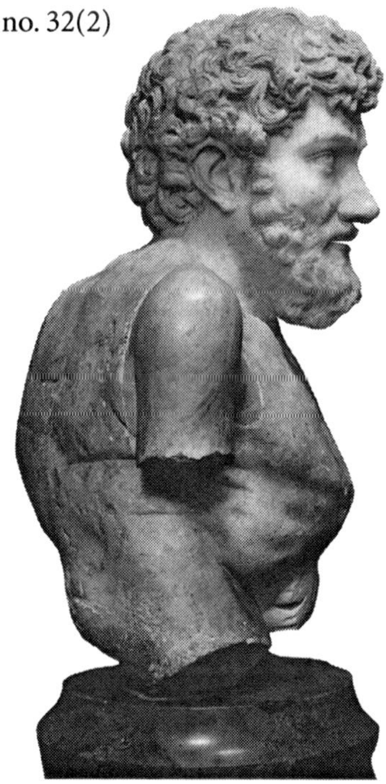

Cat. no. 33(1)

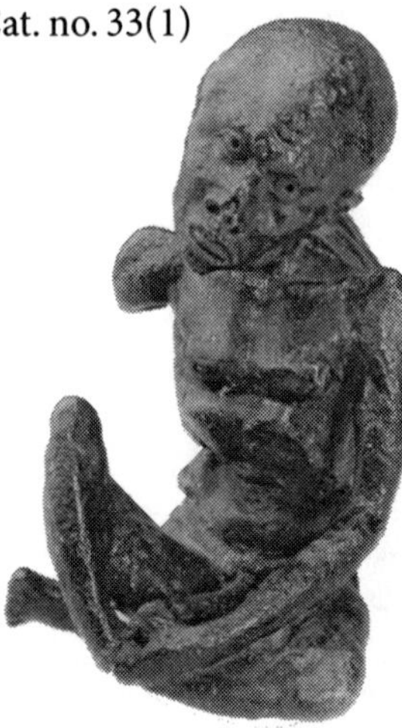

Cat. no. 33(2)

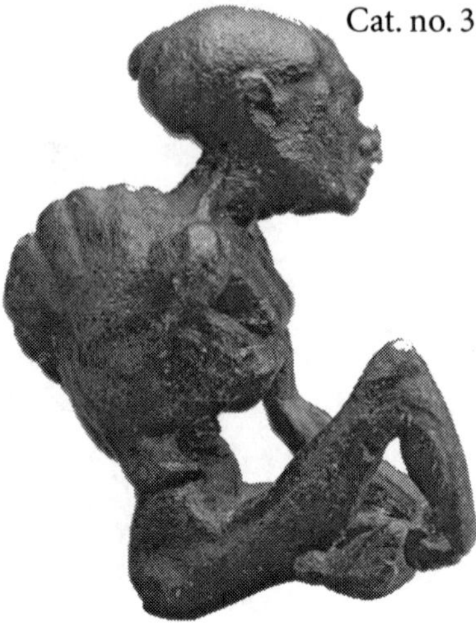

Cat. no. 34(1)

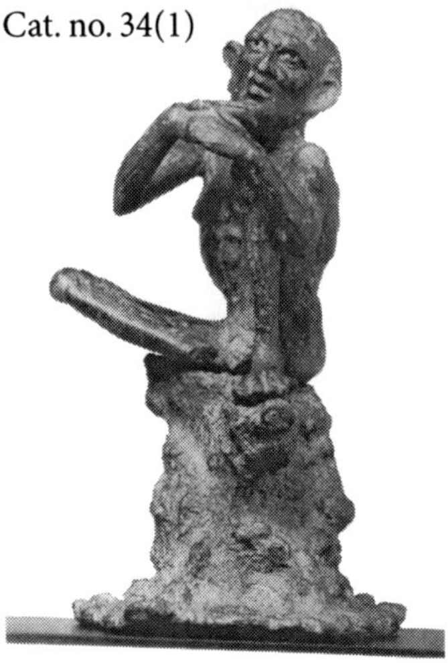

Cat. no. 34(2)

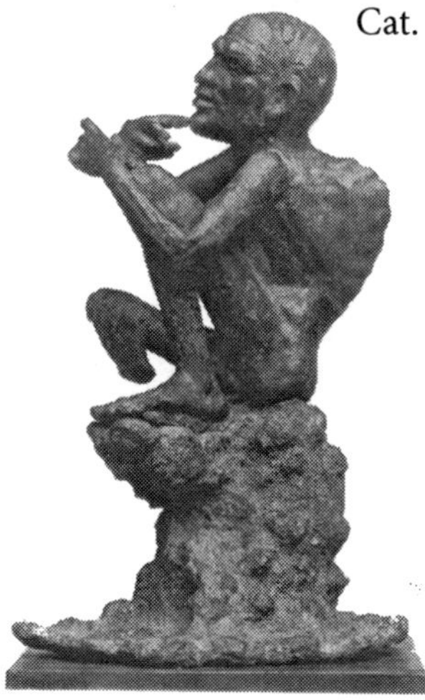

Cat. no. 35(1)

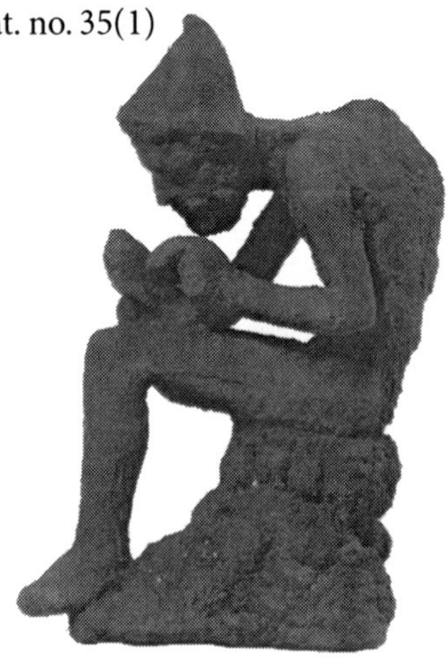

Cat. no. 35(2)

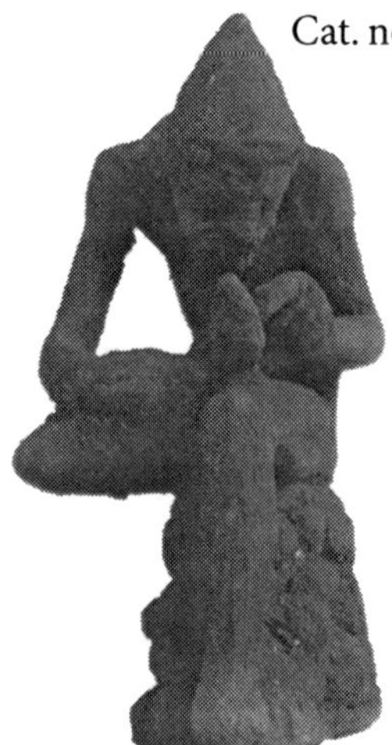

Cat. no. 36

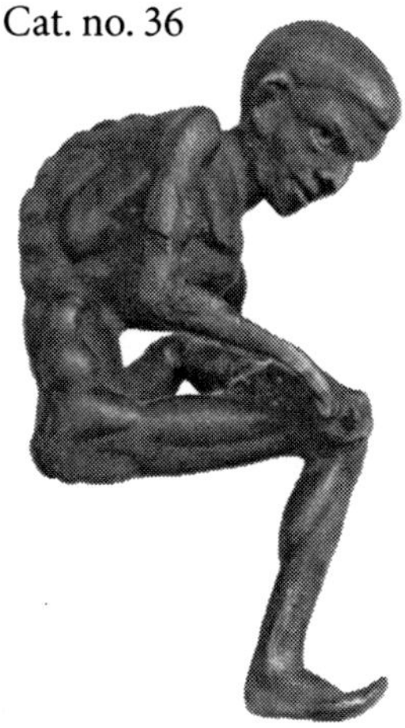

Cat. no. 37(1)

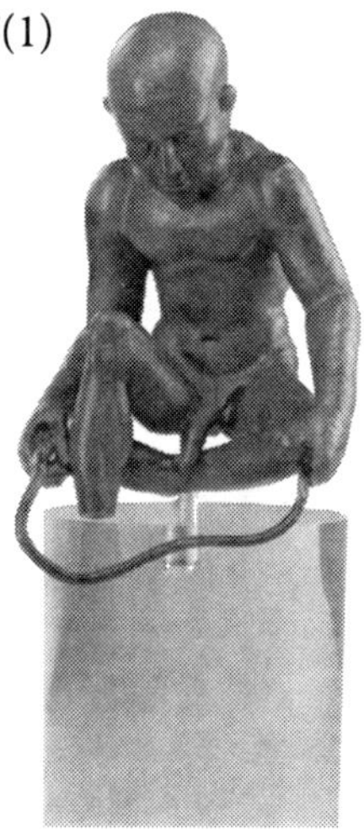

Cat. no. 37(2)

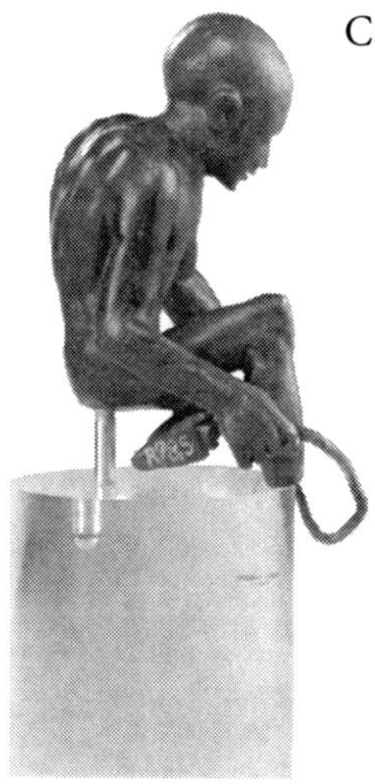

Cat. no. 40(1)

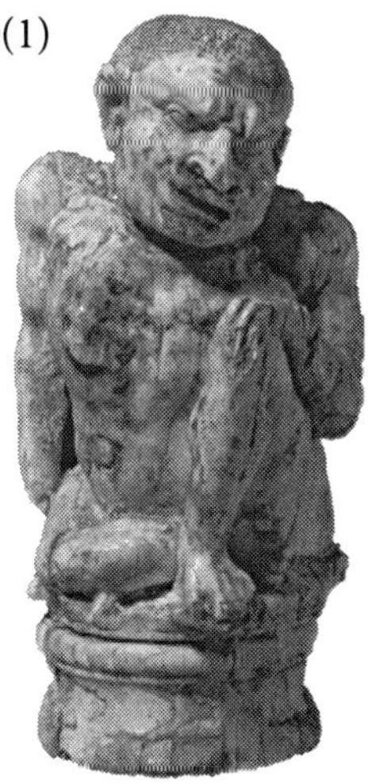

Cat. no. 40(2)

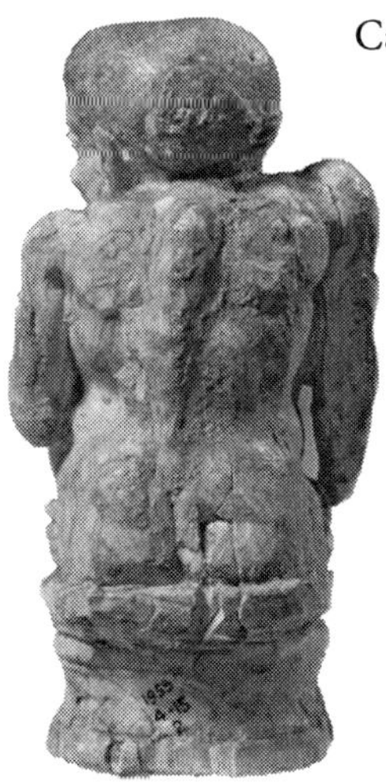

Cat. no. 41

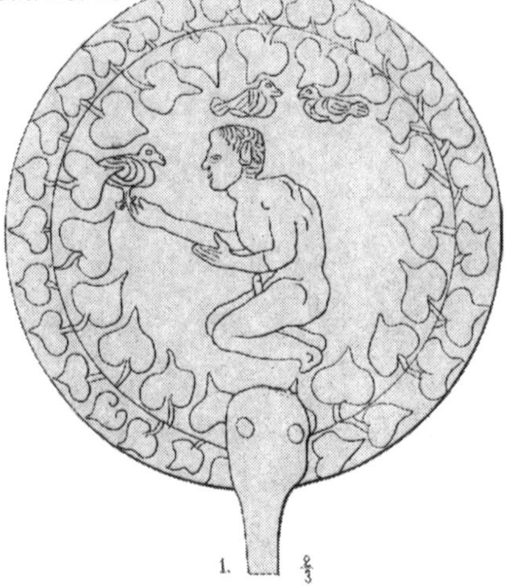

Cat. no. 44

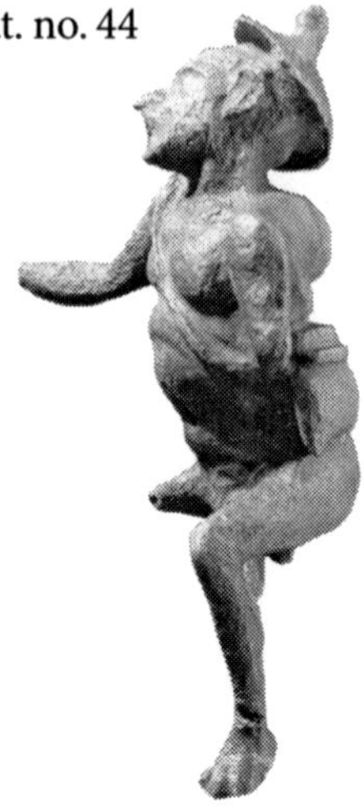

Cat. no. 45(1)

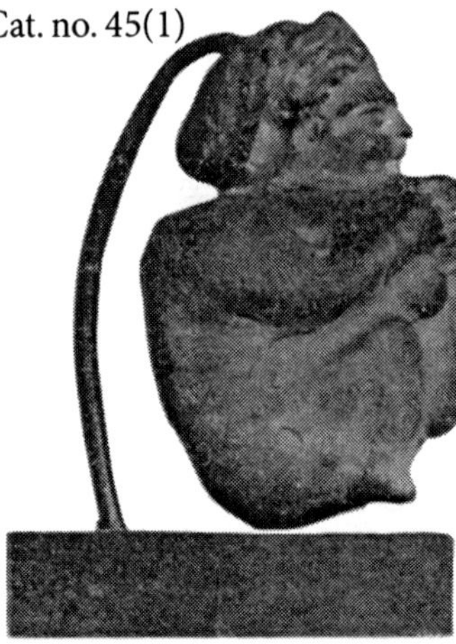

Cat. no. 45(2)

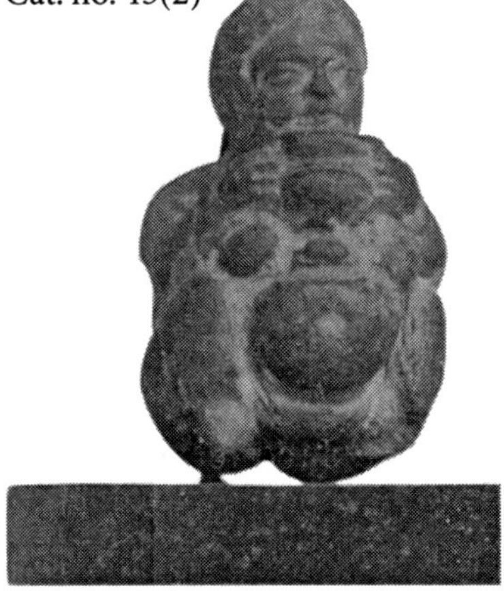

Cat. no. 46

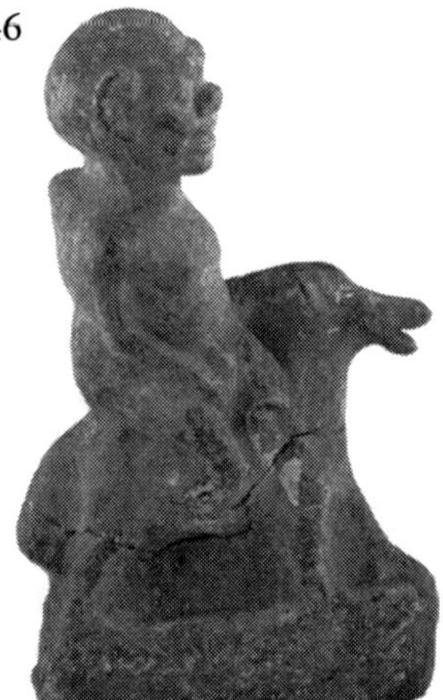

Cat. no. 48(1)

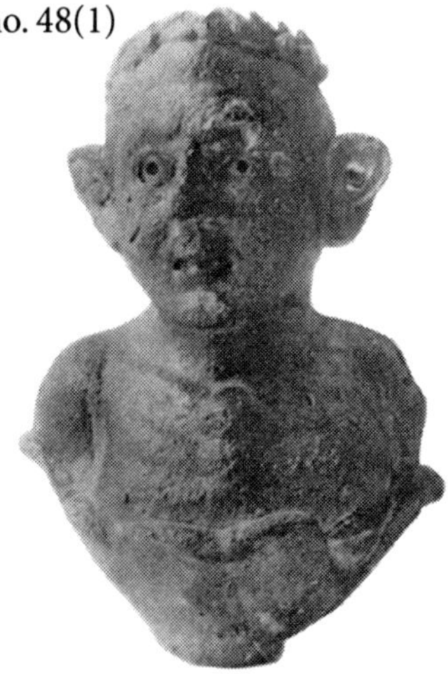

Cat. no. 48(2)

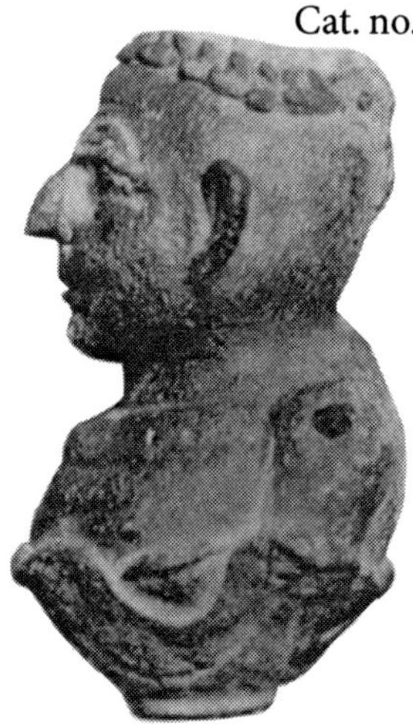

Cat. no. 50

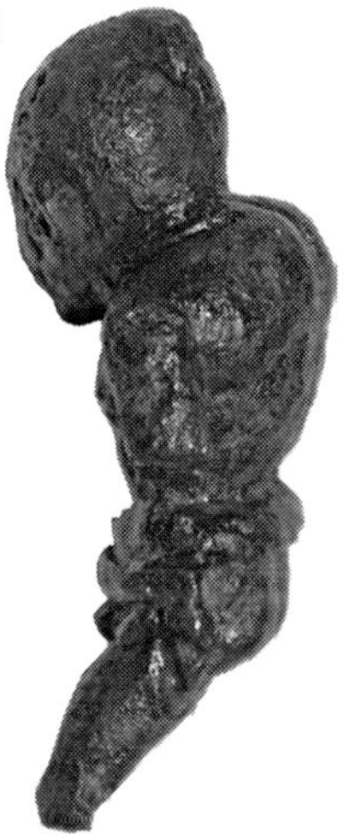

Cat. no. 52

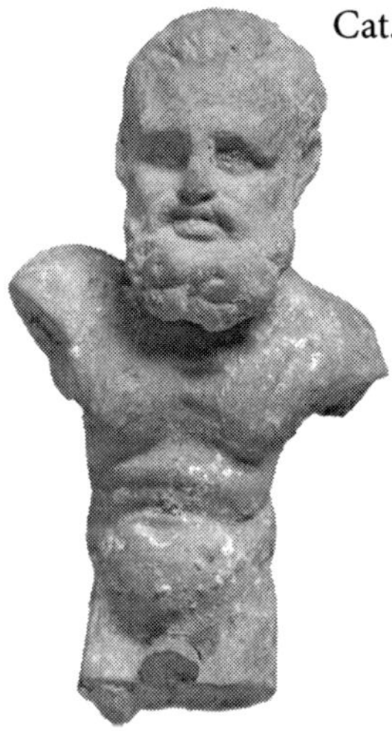

Cat. no. 55(1)

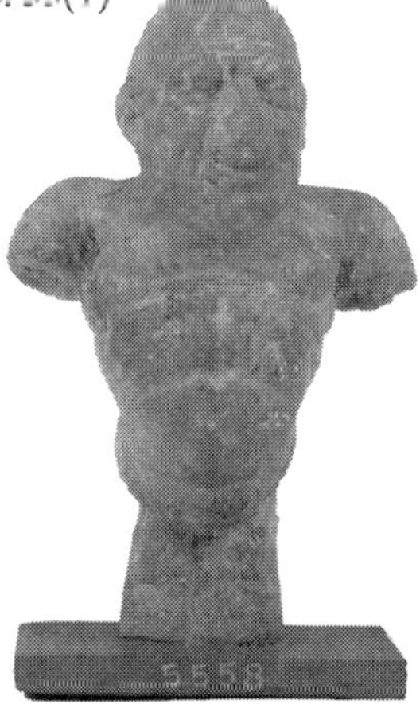

Cat. no. 55(2)

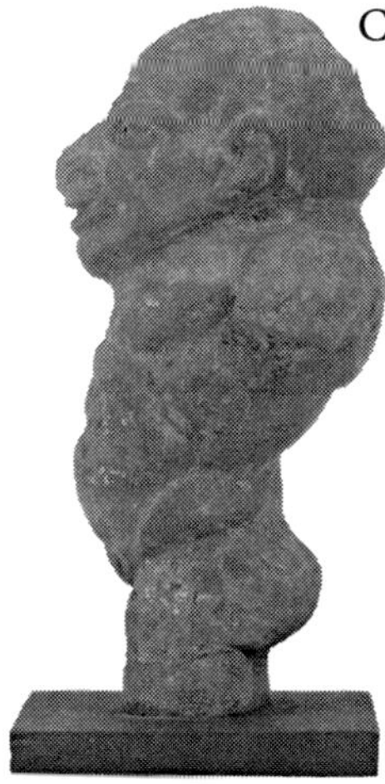

Notes

Introduction

1 See especially Stiker (1999). For individual studies on deformed and disabled bodies, see below, note 4.
2 Although this catalogue is extensive, and I have set out specific criteria for positively identifying a representation as that of a hunchback (see Chapter 1), I cannot promise to have located every representation of a hunchback in Greco-Roman antiquity. It is my hope, however, that this catalogue will become the main source of reference for future scholarly investigation and that future contributions can be made to further advance the study of the hunchback in antiquity.
3 See also Rose (1997a, 1997b, 1997c, 1998, 2003 and 2006).
4 On dwarfs, see Dasen (1993 and 2006) and also Garmaise, *Dwarfs* (1996). On hermaphrodites, see Ajootian (1988, 1990, 1995 and 1997) and also Brisson (2002). On the black African and pygmy, see Clarke (1996, 1998 and 2005a) and Versluys (2002) and Meyboom and Versluys (2005). On deafness, see Laes (2011 and 2013). On lameness, see Pestilli (2005). On obesity, see Bradley (2011), with an extensive bibliography of earlier studies. On blindness in the Roman world, see Trentin (2013b), also with an extensive bibliography including sources for the Greek world.
5 Wace, *Grotesques* (1903/4) and Stevenson, *Pathological Grotesque* (1975) provide the earliest and most extensive catalogues of hunchback representations, but these are limited to sculptural representations and exclude those that appear on two-dimensional media. Although these representations are few in number, they are nevertheless important for understanding the corpus of hunchbacks as a whole.
6 See Trentin (2009 and 2011) and Masséglia, *Body Language* (2015), especially Chapter 5, 'The Body Language of Grotesques', which includes analysis of Hellenistic representations of dwarfs and cripples (e.g. the hunchback). I am grateful to Jane Masséglia for making her monograph available to me.
7 In its modern usage, the term grotesque is synonymous with 'crude' or 'ugly'; however, these associations have little to do with its original meaning. The term

originally referred to a type of decorative painting consisting of human and animal forms, fantastically combined and interwoven with plant and architectural elements. Murals of this kind first came to light around 1500 in the course of excavations at Rome, particularly under the *Domus Aurea*. From *grotte*, Italian 'caves' and, by extension, 'excavations', came the adjective *grottesco* and the noun, *la grottesca*, denoting this type of painting. Early in the sixteenth century, however, this terminology became distorted from its original meaning. The term grotesque eventually came to include all art that was considered degenerate; anything that did not represent the ideal or the beautiful, but rather the unnatural, the fantastic, or the extremely exaggerated. For detailed studies on the grotesque in both art and literature, see Barasch (1971); Thomson (1972); Harpham (1982); Bakhtin (1984).

8 The first recognition of the pathological genre in antiquity was established by medical practitioners at the renowned medical school *La Salpêtrière* in France. Pioneers in this process included Professor Jean Martin Charcot and Dr Paul Richer, who published *Les difformes et les malades dans l'art* in 1879.

9 As medical teaching aids, see Laumonier (1946: 318); Besques (1972: 153); and Leyenaar-Plaisier (1984: 70). As prophylactic charms, see Charbonneaux (1936: 20) and Levi (1941: 220).

10 Wace, *Grotesques* (1903/4: 103–14). This remains the most widely recognized interpretation for their function. The hunchback as apotropaion will be fully explored in Chapter 3.

11 Richter, *Grotesques* (1913: 154). Richter argued that the 'whole varied class of grotesques' (p. 151) functioned as mimes, using one example, the hunchback now in New York (cat. no. 8), as evidence for this assertion. Bieber (1961: 248) supported this, at least in part, stating, 'The actors of the farce were often people with abnormally ugly bodies, extremely lean and small or excessively tall or fat for comic contrast.' Other scholars have also recognized mimic actors in *some* representations, e.g. Stevenson, *Pathological Grotesque* (1975) and Barton (1993). For a more recent evaluation of Richter's mime interpretation, see Masséglia, *Body Language* (2015), Appendix 1.

12 For the various interpretations, see: Perdrizet (1911: 58), who suggests that some grotesques were votives to Asclepius; Binsfeld (1956: 43–4), who suggests that they were considered comical as well as apotropaic; Shapiro (1984: 391–2), who argues that the attribution of a large or erect phallus is an indication of sexual potency; Giuliani (1987), who argues that they served as sympotic entertainment; Wrede (1988), who suggests that they had Dionysian associations; Barton (1993), who suggests that they were court pets, as well as mimers and talismans; and Fischer and Zachman (1994: 70–3), who suggest that they were cultic, but also served as talismans.

Chapter 1

1 See Ruffer (1910: 176, plate IV, figure 2); Bieber (1961: 96); Fowler (1989: 67). The Metropolitan Museum identifies the figure as a dwarf and not a hunchback.

2 These include: cat. no. 3, from Egypt; cat. no. 7, from Egypt; cat. no. 8, from the Esquiline in Rome; cat. no. 9, from Cairo; cat. no. 10, from Smyrna; cat. no. 16, from Pompeii; cat. no. 17, from a Roman villa in Jekmejeh; cat. no. 18, from Cologne; cat. no. 20, from a Roman villa in the Rhône Valley; cat. no. 21, from Egypt; cat. no. 22, from Egypt; cat. no. 23, from Strasbourg; cat. no. 24, from Egypt; cat. no. 30, from Smyrna; cat. no. 32, from the Baths of Caracalla in Rome; cat. no. 34, from Rome; cat. no. 35, from Alexandria; cat. no. 37, from a Roman villa in Herbrechtingen; cat. no. 40, from Egypt; cat. no. 41, from Tarquinia; cat. no. 44, from Egypt; cat. no. 45, from Cyprus; cat. no. 48, from Egypt; cat. no. 49, from Alexandria; cat. no. 51, from Egypt; and cat. nos 52–5, from Smyrna.

3 These include: cat. no. 16, discovered in Pompeii; cat. no. 17, from a Roman villa in Jekmejeh, near Antioch; cat. no. 18, from the Hahnentor area in Cologne; cat. no. 20, from a Roman villa in the Rhône Valley; cat. no. 23, from a villa under the Rue du Vieux Marché aux Vins in Strasbourg; cat. no. 32, from the Baths of Caracalla in Rome; and cat. no. 37, from a Roman villa near Herbrechtingen, Stuttgart.

4 This wall painting is reproduced in *Le Antichità di Ercolano Esposte*, Tomo 7, LXVII, p. 299, though notably, the erect penis of the hunchback pygmy was expurgated. Helbig (1868: 381, no. 1539), who gives precise provenances when they exist, just gives 'P.' for 'Pompeii'.

5 For a detailed analysis of this sculpture and its (mis)identification as Aesop, see Trentin (2009).

6 The emaciation of some of these figures is often associated with famine and disease, though some scholars have seen these figures as personifications of envy, whose characteristic features include self-strangulation, emaciation, pallor, sunken eyes, an angry brow and a hunched back. See Dunbabin (1986) and Dunbabin and Dickie (1983). Those figures with side- or top-knots of hair may sport the *cirrus* hairstyle, characteristic of career boxers and pankratiasts. In his catalogue of Hellenistic and Roman representations of dwarfs, Garmaise, *Dwarfs*, 110, describes eleven figurines of dwarfs as possessing knots or tufts of hair on the top of their heads. Brunet (2003), however, has recognized only two of these as clearly having a top-knot. According to Brunet (2003: 20, footnote 12), what Garmaise took to be a tuft of hair is rather a lip that allows these figurines to be used as containers for holding oil or perfume, or may have served as an attachment for a chain. In

representations of the hunchback, it is unclear whether these tufts of hair represent the *cirrus* hairstyle or the lip. On the *cirrus*, see Gassowska (1966: 421–7); Brunet (2003: 18–20).

7 So according to Perdrizet (1911) and Picard (1958).

8 These sticks have been variously interpreted: Levi, *Lucky Hunchback*, 228 argued that they were magic sticks, 'held in such a way as to present their tips pointing in all directions, thus ready to act whether the Evil Eye attacks from above or from below, from the right or from the left'. Goldman (1943: 22), who follows Jahn (1857), argued that they were 'clappers' used by dancers. Masséglia, *Body Language* identifies them as rhythm sticks. Both suggestions suggest that they serve the same purpose: they functioned as talismans by making noise and thus frightening the evil eye. The identification of rhythm sticks follows that of Masséglia, *Body Language*.

9 Cat. nos 34 and 35 sit on rocks and it is likely that cat. no. 33 was similarly represented, as noted by Jantzen (1958: 49).

10 Perdrizet (1911: 60) suggests that the figure's crown is similar to that worn by individuals attending the sacrifice and banquet as part of the Eleusinian Mysteries at Alexandria; supporting evidence for this is limited, however, and as such this association must remain purely speculative.

11 For a full description of the physical features that characterize the black African, see Snowden (1970: 5–11). On the role of the black African in ancient art and literature, see also Thompson (1989) and Clarke (1996, 1998). For a full description of the iconographic conventions used to characterize the dwarf, see Dasen, *Dwarfs*, 165–74 and on the pygmy, see Versluys (2002) and Meyboom and Versluys (2005). On the role of the dwarf in ancient art and literature, see also Garmaise, *Dwarfs*. Clarke (1998: 122) states that it is not difficult to distinguish between the pygmy and the Aethiops; however, both Spinazzola (1953) and Maiuri (1956) characterize several black Africans on mosaics in Pompeii as pygmies. Presumably ancient audiences would also have found the blurring in iconography problematic too for identification.

12 On this perfect and ageless body, see Spivey (1996); A. F. Stewart (1990); P. Stewart (1997).

13 Bieber (1961: 97) and Pollitt (1986: 138) both suggest that the figures were religious dancers but Pollitt also notes that they may have been caricatures. The dwarfs illustrated in Figure 3 are those from the Mahdia shipwreck. On the symbolism of their iconography and their function and meaning, see Wrede (1988); Pfisterer-Haas (1994); Garmaise, *Dwarfs*; Fischer (1998) and Masséglia, *Body Language*.

14 For an explanation of the different types of dances and the meaning of the positioning of the arms, legs, head, etc., see Emmanuel (1916); Prudhommeau (1965).

15 There are seven extant representations of the Aphrodite Kallipygos type catalogued in the *Lexicon Iconographicum Mythologiae Classicae* (*LIMC*) II.1 (1984) 85–6, nos 765–71. The type is associated with a story in Athenaeus' *Deipnosophists* 12.554 c–e in which two peasant girl sisters from Syracuse become involved in a dispute as to which one has the more beautiful buttocks and enlist the help of a young man who happens to pass by. The sisters later dedicate a temple to Aphrodite Kallipygos. The religious cult of Aphrodite Kallipygos at Syracuse is also mentioned by Clement of Alexandria, *Protrepticus* 2.39.2. Controversy has long raged as to whether the figure actually represents Aphrodite at all, or rather, a dancer, courtesan or ordinary maiden.

16 Indeed, modern psycho-sociological theory suggests that 'abnormality arouses in some "normal" beholders, a temptation to go beyond looking to knowing, in the full carnal sense, the ultimate other' (Fiedler 1978: 137).

17 Palazzo dei Conservatori, Rome, MC1186. For dating and status of the sculpture, see Zanker (1974); Haskell and Penny (1981: no. 78). For the reception of the sculpture in the Renaissance and beyond, see Cocke (1980).

18 British Museum, London, 1755. See Kapossy (1969: 45); Masséglia, *Body Language*.

19 Staatliche Museum, Berlin, 8626. See Smith (1991: 137); Masséglia, *Body Language*.

20 Smith (1991: 137) suggests that the thorn-in-foot motif serves to connect the Spinario to the ideal countryside of the Dionysian world. Onians (1979: 128) associates the theme, especially in group compositions, with the wounding power of Eros, citing Theocritus' *Idyll* IV (55) as evidence. Do the lone Spinario figures also make oblique statements about the wounding power of love? Can we read the hunchback Spinario in an eroticized context? See Chapter 3.

21 Beardsley (1929: 37–8) and Havelock (1971: 136) have regarded the statuette as comical, 'a parody of the dignified original', whereas Higgins (1967: 120) has described it as 'a sympathetic study of a racial type'.

22 Masséglia, *Body Language*, Chapter 4, 'The Body Language of "Genre" Figures', and her discussion of rustic peasants.

Chapter 2

1 All catalogue numbers except 16, 17, 20, 32, and 41.

2 The visual representation of non-elite or 'ordinary' Romans is thoroughly explored by Clarke (2003), though his focus is on wall paintings and mosaic pavements. A similar approach to the miniature is adopted here.

3 Over the past decade there has been some attempt to re-configure the hierarchy of ancient art. Most influential in the rise of the miniature has been Bartman, *Miniature*. Bartman presents the first scholarly exploration devoted entirely to the miniature, albeit in terms of the miniature copy. Her analysis begins with a general discussion of the history and function of the miniature and is followed by case studies devoted to several famous statuary types: the Resting Satyr, the Lateran Poseidon, the *Herakles Epitrapezos*. These case studies consider the techniques, formal values, and meanings of the miniature while providing methodological models for the understanding of any copy.

4 Smith (1991: 137). Smith also suggests that poverty and old age were suitable subjects for statues because they were in some ways redeemable, unlike the more awful human afflictions of disease and deformity.

5 For example, Lamb (1929: 203) states: 'in style they [grotesques] are often rough and unfinished'; and Bieber (1955: 102) characterizes Alexandrian art (where representations of grotesques were abundant) as 'not really great art'.

6 A number of important sources on bronze statuary have been used to aid in the analysis of the various techniques of manufacture and decoration. See Lamb (1929); Kozloff and Mitten (1988); and Haynes (1992).

7 Richter (1913: 149–56), who argues that the figure represents a character of the mine, states: 'the period to which the statue belongs must be late Greek; at least it is inconceivable that a work of so much spirit and animation and of such masterly technique originated in Roman times; and its style and conception do not permit an earlier dating' (p. 150). Kozloff and Mitten (1988: 166) argue that, if an actor, the figure may likely have played in a crude Atellan farce, but seems more likely to recall Etruscan images of Charun, god of the underworld. With regards to date they state, 'Given the reported Italian provenance for this bronze, it is probable that the image is a late Republican or early imperial version, likely dating to the first century BCE.'

8 Jantzen (1958: 47); Museum für Kunst und Gewerbe collection database.

9 A number of important sources on terracotta statuettes have been used to aid in the analysis of the different regional styles and techniques of manufacture and decoration. See especially Uhlenbrock (1990).

10 Garland, *Beholder*, 117: 'The misshapen body and head, the twisted facial features, the contorted yet highly naturalistic pose, and the expression of painful resignation, all combine to make this one of the most haunting works in the entire repertoire of grotesques.'

11 See Chapter 1, note 2.

12 These seven are: cat. no. 16, which depicts a wall painting discovered in Pompeii; cat. no. 17, which depicts a mosaic pavement decorating a Roman villa in Jekmejeh,

near Antioch; cat. no. 18, which depicts a bronze statuette from the Hahnentor area in Cologne; cat. no. 20, which depicts a vase found at a Roman villa in the Rhône Valley; cat. no. 23, which depicts a bronze statuette from Strasbourg, in a villa under the Rue du Vieux Marché aux Vins; cat. no. 33, which depicts a large-scale marble statue from the Baths of Caracalla in Rome; and cat. no. 37, which depicts a bronze statuette from a Roman villa near Herbrechtingen, Stuttgart.

13 On Roman bronzes from the provinces, see Reinach (1894), Boucher (1973), and Oggiano-Bitar (1984).

14 Numerous small-scale statuettes have been recovered in these areas, occasionally *in situ*, thus supplying important evidence for the function of the miniature. For Delos, see Marcadé (1969); for Priene, see Rumscheid (2006); for Pergamon, see Boehringer and Pinkwart (1967); for Pompeii, see Tronchin (2011).

15 That is not to say, however, that miniature works of art were exclusively private in function, nor monumental works exclusively public in function. Indeed, the division between monumental and miniature display spaces was often blurred, and, in some instances, both miniature and monumental were displayed alongside one another, creating dynamic visual ensembles. These ensembles often worked to confound a viewer's expectations, both in their choice of subject matter and in how they manipulated and related monumental against miniature. See Bartman, *Miniature*.

16 Bartman, *Miniature*; see Chapter 3, pp. 39–42 for a summary of the possibilities for display of the miniature.

17 For the display of terracotta figurines from Priene, see Rumscheid (2006: 60).

18 See Bartman, *Miniature*, 41. For the use of stone tables in antiquity, see the doctoral theses of Cohon (1984) and Moss (1988).

19 Jantzen (1958: 49) states that 'We can safely assume that the Hamburg hunchback (cat. no. 32) sat on an equivalent rocky base to the Berlin hunchback.'

20 As Jashemski and Macdougall (1981) and Jashemski (1987) have demonstrated, ancient Roman villa gardens were elaborately decorated with sculpture, both large- and small scale, and the natural and man-made garden landscape was manipulated to create dynamic visual ensembles.

21 Over 135 representations of Hermaphroditus have been catalogued by Ajootian in the *Lexicon Iconographicum Mythologiae Classicae* (LIMC) VII (1990). Ajootian (268–85) divides 'Hermaphroditos reclining' into two groups: 'Hermaphroditos recumbent on stomach' and 'Hermaphroditos recumbent on back'. The statuette from the House of Octavius Quartio is recumbent on its back, but exhibits the characteristic exposed genitalia of the Hermaphroditus '*anasyromenos*' type, also catalogued by Ajootian (1995: 275).

22 For a full description of the statuette, see Spinazzola (1953: 657); Nappo (1998: 50–51); and Tronchin (2011: 39–40).

23 Von Stackelberg (2009), Tronchin (2011). Von Stackelberg (2009: 5) interprets the garden 'as an active space of movement and memory' and uses the House of Octavius Quartio as a case study to understand the messages communicated to visitors via garden space and sculpture. Tronchin (2011: 35) 'position[s] the decorative ensemble of this house into larger patters of cultural phenomena such as Egyptomania, copy–model relationships, the economics of sculpture production, and assertion of *Romanitas*'. She concludes that the sculpture in the House of Octavius Quartio not only reflected personal tastes, but also played a role in affirming the owner's status within the community of Pompeian elite (p. 47).

24 A relief now in Ince Blundell Hall in England, dating to the first century BC, unequivocally connects the Spinario with a rural setting: the Spinario sits on a rock next to a tree in the company of Orpheus and satyrs. See Ashmole (1929: pl. 45).

25 British Museum, London, 1755. See Kapossy (1969: 45); Masséglia, *Body Language*; and the collection database of the British Museum website, with more information and relevant bibliography.

26 Staatliche Museum, Berlin, 8626. See Smith (1991: 137); Rumscheid (1998: 145); Masséglia, *Body Language*.

27 Masséglia, *Body Language*, Chapter 4, 'The Body Language of "Genre" Figures' in the section on 'Fishermen and Peasants'.

28 On viewer integration in Hellenistic sculpture, see von Hesberg (1988) and Zanker (2004). The Romans also fully exploited the concept of viewer integration.

29 As I have analysed this statue at length elsewhere (see Trentin, 2009), discussing its history, the problems of its identification, and its place in the Baths, the analysis here focuses solely on a viewer's optic and haptic encounter with this hunchback.

30 Figure 6 is an engraving of the original sculpture with its semi-erect penis, after Visconti (1811: pl. 12). Stevenson (1975: 238, no. 46) notes that the Albani Torlonia bust had a 'prominent phallus, expurgated from most photographs'. Bol (1989: 227) states that it was sometime in the eighteenth century when the phallus was removed and covered by the fig leaf.

31 For those few hunchbacks represented with a portrait-style head, see cat. nos 9, 17, 32, 48, 49 and 52.

32 On the sculptural programme of the Baths and viewer engagement, see Marvin (1983) and Trentin (2009: 145–51).

33 Touching statues in public baths may not have been so uncouth: Bradley (2009b: 441) has shown that the famous Hellenistic bronze statue of a bruised and battered seated boxer, once set up at the Baths of Constantine in Rome, now on display at the Museo Nazionale Romano – Palazzo Massimo alle Terme (inv. 1055), shows

signs of wearing on his hands and right foot, evidence that it was frequently touched (for inspiration?) by passers-by in the Baths.

34 For the (mis)identification of this hunchback as the famous Greek fabulist Aesop, see Trentin (2009: 134–9).

35 In her book, *On Longing*, Stewart (1984) argues (within the broader context of literary theory) that all miniaturization is essentially a means of domestication, and moreover, that in the miniaturization of the Other there is evidence of an impulse to know and to dominate the unknown. See Chapter 2, 'The Miniature,' pp. 37–69 and Chapter 4, 'The Imaginary Body,' pp. 104–31.

36 Representations of dwarfs provide the most copious evidence for this phenomenon. Dasen, *Dwarfs* has examined the frequency with which dwarfs were represented in Greek art, depicted in a variety of roles, from personal attendants to paidagogoi, but, as Garmaise, *Dwarfs*, 56–93, and more recently Dasen (2013) and Masséglia, *Body Language*, Chapter 4, have shown, it was not until the Hellenistic period and beyond that ('real-life' and representational) dwarfs became popular as entertainers. The same is true for the hunchback.

37 Plut. *Mor.* 520c.

38 Quint. *Inst.* 2.5.11.

39 For the popularity of deformed slaves, especially in the Roman imperial court, see Trentin (2011).

40 Lucian, *Symp.* 18.

41 Plin. *NH* 34.6.

42 SHA, *Comm.* 11.2. For a full analysis of this troubling episode, see Trentin (2011).

43 Masséglia, *Body Language*, Chapter 4, 'The Body Language of "Grotesques"'.

44 Emmanuel (1916: 79–99, figs 88–181) describes and illustrates numerous positions of the arms in the various types of ancient (Greek) dances.

45 Dieterich (1897) believes the scene represented Dionysiac revellers. The existence of entertaining troupes in antiquity is well documented. According to Xenophon (*Symp.* 2.1, 8, 11, 14) a Syracusan manager trained slaves and freedmen in the arts of professional entertainers and hired his troupe. Managers must surely have realized that the presence of deformed individuals would have increased the interest of their shows.

46 The iconography, context and distribution of Nilotic scenes has been systematically studied by Versluys (2002) and Meyboom and Versluys (2005). For this particular representation, see Versluys (2002: 211–12).

Chapter 3

1 See cat. nos 1–5, 7, 10, 12–17, 20–26, 28, 30–33, 35, 39–41, 48.

2 See Dover (1978: esp. 127) for differences in representation of penises and phalluses.

3 As recognized by Wace, *Grotesques*, 103–14; Levi (1941: 220–32); Binsfeld (1956); Barton (1993: 91–8); Dasen, *Dwarfs*, 1–3, 10–11.

4 Some of the most thorough sources on the superstition of the Evil Eye in antiquity are Jahn (1855), Elworthy (1895) and Seligmann (1922). More recent is Dunbabin and Dickie (1983).

5 On the apotropaic use of the phallus, see Jahn (1855: 28–110); Herter (1932); Slane and Dickie (1993: 483–505); Orrells (2005).

6 See Wace, *Grotesques*; Levi, *Lucky Hunchback*; Dickie (1996); Clarke (2007a) and Masséglia, *Body Language*.

7 Plut. *Quaest. conviv.* 5.7, 681–2 asserts that the strangeness of apotropaea draws the eyes of the envious away from the objects needing protection. This has led scholars to argue that the physical appearance of deformed individuals was intended to arouse laughter or shame and thus divert the attention of the envious. See Levi (1941 and 1947) and Clarke (1998 and 2007a).

8 Planudes Manuscript 1 of the *Life of Aesop*. See the next note for more information on the *Life*.

> *ἐτύγχανε δ' ὢν οὐ μόνον δοῦλος ἀλλὰ καὶ δυσειδέστατα τῶν ἐπ' αὐτοῦ πάντων ἀνθρώπων εἶχε. καὶ γὰρ φοξὸς ἦν, σιμὸς τὴν ῥῖνα, σιμὸς τὸν τράχηλον, πρόχειλος, μέλας – ὅθεν καὶ τοῦ ὀνόματος ἔτυχε ταὐτὸν γὰρ Ἀἴσωπος τῷ Αἰθίοπι – προγάστωρ, βλαισός καὶ κυφός . . .*
>
> He was not only a slave but the ugliest of all men of his time. He had a pointy head, a snub nose, a snub neck, thick lips and dark skin – from which he got his name, for 'Aesop' means the same as 'Ethiopian' – was pot-bellied, stunted and hunchbacked.

9 The *Life of Aesop* is largely considered a 'biographical romance' by Lissarrague (2000: 132) and a 'satirical fiction' by Hopkins (1993: 10). It survives in at least fifteen manuscripts and four papyrus fragments, all of which have been edited by Perry (1952). The oldest and most complete text of the *Life* is contained in a tenth century manuscript in the library of J. P. Morgan, New York, and is based on an archetype composed or re-written between 100 BCE and 200 CE. As a historical figure, Aesop is enigmatic, but as a legendary figure he is important 'for reflecting on notions of identity and alterity in the ancient Greek world' (Lissarrague 2000: 132).

10 Perry (1936: 40), Morgan Manuscript 16. Translation from Dickie (1995: 242).

11 Perry (1936: 83). Westermann Text 16. Translation from Dickie (1995: 242).

12 Poll. *Onom.* 7.108–9:

> *πρὸ δὲ τῶν χαμίνων τοῖς χαλχεῦσιν ἔθος ἦν γελοῖᾳ τ ινα καταρτᾶν ἢ ἐπιπλάττειν ἐπὶ φθόνου ἀποτροπῇ ˙ἐχαλεῖτο δὲ βασκάνια ὡς χαὶ Ἀριστοφᾴνης λέγει.*

> Aristophanes fragment 607 PCG:

> *πλὴν εἴ τις πρίαιτο δεό μενος*
> *βασκάνιον ἐπικάμινον ἀ νδρὸς χαλκέως*

13 Phrynicus, *Praep. soph.* p. 53.6–10 Borries: *ἀνθρποειδὲς κατασκεύασμα βραχὺ παρηλλαγμένον τὴν ἀνθρωπείαν φύσιν τοῦ μὴ βασκαίνεσθαι αὐτῶν ἐργασίαν*

14 A variety of physical features were regarded in antiquity as characteristic of images of envy, including physical distortions such as emaciation and a humped back and actions that represent the *phthoneros* strangling himself or chocking, characterized by the gesture of the hands clutched to the throat.

15 See Giuliani (1987: 718–20, fig. 18); and Mitchell (2013: 285, fig. 10).

16 The main ruins of the villa consist of a pool surrounded on all sides by colonnaded porticoes and decorated with geometric mosaic pavements. A vestibule beyond the west end of the north portico yielded the only three figural mosaics of the complex; it is here that our hunchback mosaic was discovered. The villa, and its decorative mosaics, have been thoroughly analysed, especially with regards to their apotropaic significance, by Levi (1941, 1947).

17 See Chapter 1, note 8.

18 The phrases *καὶ σύ*, *καὶ σοί*, or *et tibi*, *et tibi sit* often appear in association with single phalluses, phallic monsters or men with phalluses and function as threats or curses. For examples, see Slane and Dickie (1993: 490–2, esp. footnote 44); and Levi, *Lucky Hunchback*, 225–6.

19 Slane and Dickie (1993) suggest that the phrase is to be read as a prophylactic curse; however, Cimok (2000: 34) suggests that the phrase could simply be a warning to visitors of the house. Levi, *Lucky Hunchback*, 226 notes that the *καὶ σύ* formulation also appears in contexts of well-wishes, and could have been intended to have a benevolent purpose.

20 See Arist. *IA*, 11: all children are dwarf-like.

21 Levi, *Lucky Hunchback*, 220–25 explains in detail the apotropaic significance of each of these animals and weapons and provides numerous examples of their use on monuments elsewhere.

22 In the earliest publication of this mosaic, Levi identified this figure as a dwarf. Since then, however, others (e.g. Clarke 2007a and Mitchell 2013) have mistakenly identified him as a hunchbacked dwarf. The figure does not possess a visible hump,

as clearly represented in the mosaic beneath, and although a reading of this figure as a hunchback would certainly add explicit evidence for the hunchback as apotropaion, it remains, nevertheless, a dwarf.

23 Slane and Dickie (1993: 491) suggest that two more phalluses emerge from either side of the dwarf's head and also point towards the eye; however, Levi, who first publishes the mosaic, does not make this observation. Although there does seem to be at least one object protruding from the dwarf's head, I am not convinced that this is a phallus.

24 Masséglia, *Body Language*: see Chapter 4, 'The Body Language of "Grotesques"'.

25 On the role of the cock in fertility and eroticism in classical antiquity, see Baird (1981–83).

26 For the excavations of necropoli at Tarquinia and the mirrors found there, see Carpino (2008).

27 The category of ivy-leaf wreath mirrors is characterized by minimal decorative elements; there are often empty spaces between the characters and the surrounding garland, as evidenced in our mirror. For the analysis of the decorative elements on Etruscan mirrors, see Wiman (1990: 105–9).

28 See especially Clarke on the Aethiops (1996, 1998); and Lissarrague on the satyr (1990a).

29 Such evidence is particularly pronounced in Latin literature: e.g. Elagabalus is said to have searched out men with large penises so that he could enjoy their affections (SHA, *Heliogab.* 5.3). Moreover, it was the exceptionally large penises of Martial's smooth-skinned attendants at the baths that attracted Philomusus and the exposure of Giton's oversized penis that caused a huge crowd to surround him with applause (Martial, *Epigr.* 11.63). Seneca describes a certain Hostius Quadra as a *monstrum* or *portentum* because he used to tour the public baths looking for the man with the largest sexual organ. This same Hostius is also said to have undergone sodomy in a room with enlarging mirrors in order to take pleasure in the false size of his partner's penis by pretending that it was really that big (Sen. *Q Nat.* 1.16.2).

30 See Helbig (1868: 381 no. 1539) and note 4 in Chapter 1.

31 See Meyboom and Versluys (2005: 170–208) for the meaning of dwarfs in Nilotic scenes.

32 Though this last feature has been expurgated from the eighteenth-century drawing. See Chapter 1, note 4

33 As recognized by Versluys (2002: 282) and Meyboom and Versluys (2005: 183).

34 See especially Clarke (2005a and 1998); Dasen, *Dwarfs* and 'pygmaioi' in *LIMC* VII; and Versluys (2002) and Meyboom and Versluys (2005).

35 Jantzen (1958: 47–51) suggests that the hunchback may have originally been seated on a rock.

36 Perry (1952: 95), Westermann Text 75–76. Translation kindly provided by Lynn Kozak.
37 Plin. *NH* 34.6.12. Loeb translation.
38 For a full analysis of this tomb, and its relationship to the passage in Pliny, see Bodel (1989).
39 See, for example: Trimalchio, *Satyricon*, or Lucian, *Onos*. See also Garland, *Beholder*, 52, on the erotic appeal of deformed slaves. It also seems to have been common to accuse the emperor of such relations with his deformed slaves. An interesting anecdote in Juvenal, *Satire X*, 309 states: 'No misshapen youth was ever unsexed by a cruel tyrant in his castle; never did Nero have a bandy-legged or scrofulous favourite, or one that was hump-backed or pot-bellied!' Juvenal's comment is presumably dependent on the fact that most readers would have been aware of Nero's unusual sexual habits; the 'unsexing' of a deformed individual was simply one more perversion to add to the list. See Trentin (2011).
40 On the practice of infibulation in antiquity, see Stieda (1902); Dingwall (1925).
41 Suetonius, *Galba* 3.3: . . . *quanquam brevi corpore atque etiam gibber*.
42 Suetonius, *Galba* 3.4.

Chapter 4

1 Scholarship on the human body in art is vast and continually growing. Studies are often grouped according to specific time periods, cultures, and/or artists. For a thorough bibliography of the most significant contributions, see the 'Preface' section under 'Further Reading' in Squire (2011: 202–5).
2 See 'Chapter III' under 'Further Reading' in Squire (2011: 213–18).
3 Perusing the standard textbooks on Greek and Roman art is here illuminating: for Greek art, see Stewart (1990) and Spivey (1996); for Roman art, see Kleiner (1992) and Ramage and Ramage (2008).
4 For the Greeks, self-control, particularly the control of one's limbs and bodily gestures, was a cardinal virtue, manifested in *sophrosyne*; the same was true for the Romans, who characterized the *vir bonus* as the good man who spoke (and acted) well. For the Greeks and *sophrosyne*, see the classic study by North (1966). For the Romans and the *vir bonus*, see Gleason (1995) and Gunderson (2000).
5 Slaves are commonly depicted holding one knee to their chest and placing the other on the ground. Beggars are depicted in a variety of positions, either with

arms extended outward or in the near-foetal position. In Greek, the word for beggar is *πτωχός*, which literally means someone who crouches or cringes.

6 As recognized by Bremmer (1991: 26).

7 On viewing pleasure and pain in the Hellenistic period, see Chapter 6 of Zanker (2004). For more recent work on the representation of emotions in ancient art, see the edited volumes by Chaniotis (2012) and Chaniotis and Ducrey (2013).

8 Although much later in date, Synesius of Cyrene, Bishop of Ptolemais c. 410–413 CE, describes the crew of a boat from Alexandria as addressing each other by nicknames derived from some physical deformity: Synesius, *Letters*, from Hercher (1965: 640).

9 So according to Perdrizet (1911) and Picard (1958). For the interpretation of pathological grotesques as votives to Asclepius, see Potter and Wells (1985), Girardon (1993) and Charlier (2008).

10 See Himmelmann (1983). The *Lagynophoria* festival is known through a fragment in Athenaios 276A which seems to be either a biography of Queen Arsinoe or an essay about her. In the fragment, the *Lagynophoria* is explained as being a rustic festival where each celebrant eats whatever is brought to him while sitting on a bed of rushes and drinking from his own wine jug.

11 See Introduction, note 11.

12 On the role and status of actors in antiquity, especially ancient Rome, see Edwards (1993, 1997).

13 Suetonius, *Galba* 3.3: *pater consulate functus, quanquam brevi corpore atque etiam gibber modicaque in dicendo facultatis causas industrie actitavit.*

14 Macrobius, *Saturnalia* 2.4 [8].

15 Macrobius, *Saturnalia* 2.6 [3–4].

16 Suetonius, *De Grammaticis*, 9: *Vixit prope ad centesimum aetatis annum . . .*

17 Suetonius, *De Grammaticis*, 9.

18 For a summary of the mortuary evidence, see Graham (2013: 254–68) as well as earlier studies by: Buccellato et al. (2008) for evidence from the Via Collatina revealing kyphosis; Canci et al. (2005) for evidence from a necropolis close to the Nomentana Way (near Rome), revealing a case of Pott's disease; Catalano, Minozzi and Pantano (2001) for evidence from seven Imperial sites in the Roman *suburbium*, revealing high levels of physical stress to the spine; and Capasso (1999) for evidence of osteoporosis at Herculaneum.

19 Rose (2003), especially her analysis of individuals suffering from visual, speech and hearing impairments.

20 For family and community networks, in relation to accommodating disability, see Rose (2003) and Laes (2008).

21 Dunbabin (1994: 3) asks this question with regard to the lack of representations of female dwarfs in her review of Dasen, *Dwarfs*.

22 The bibliography on all aspects of women's life in antiquity is vast. For general studies on women in antiquity, see Pomeroy (1975); Peradotto and Sullivan (1984); Fantham (1994); McHardy and Marshall (2004). Rose (1998) provides a short but good introductory essay on the topic of women and physical disability in ancient Greece. She focuses specifically on the representation of deformed women in the literary record and examines their status in Greek life.

23 Hdt. *Histories* 1.196 and 5.92.

24 Although obesity is not today considered a deformity, recent statistics from the United States and the United Kingdom reveal that it can be considered a disability.

25 One example is a terracotta from the American School of Classical Studies, Athens, T97. See Thompson (1954: 90–92); Grmek and Gourevitch (1998: 178). This statuette was found in the sanctuary of Demeter at Athens, suggesting that it was a votive offering to ensure fertility. On representations of obesity in antiquity, see esp. Gourevitch (1985: 195–215); Grmek and Gourevitch (1987, 1998: 165–83).

26 This goes back to prehistoric times, e.g. the numerous 'Venus' figurines dating to the early Paleolithic period, such as the 'Venus of Willendorf' in the Naturhistorisches Museum, Vienna, 7.8.1908. One theory suggests that these were fertility charms to encourage pregnancy. For this and other theories, see Rice (1982); Russel (1998); Cohen (2003).

27 Garland, *Beholder* (2010: 120). He argues this based on limited osteo-archaeological evidence which demonstrates that Greek women were short and stocky; cf. Grmek (1989, esp. 110ff.).

28 On the representation of old age in antiquity, both in art and literature, see Richardson (1933); Falkner and Luce (1989). More recent work has emerged on old age, particularly in the Roman world; see Cokayne (2003) and Parkin (2003).

29 Glyptothek, Munich, 437. A similar version is held at the Capitoline Museums, Rome, MC299. See Furtwängler and Wolters (1910); Waldhauer (1946). This sculpture was originally thought to depict the celebrated statue which Pliny the Elder (Plin. *NH* 36.32) ascribes to a certain Myron, though this attribution has been refuted.

30 Pollitt (1986: 9, 143) suggests that this specific wine jug might also connote the *Lagynophoria*. Smith (1991: 138) suggests that this statue might have been a votive connected with such a festival.

31 Two representations closely connected to the Drunken Old Woman include the so-called 'New York Old Market Woman' in the Metropolitan Museum of Art, New York, 9.39, and the head of a 'Laughing Old Woman' in the Staatliche Kunstsammlungen, Dresden, 475. Both women also appear to be associated with the Dionysian world, indicated by the ivy wreaths on their heads. A useful study on the iconography of all these images and their dating is Sande (1995).

Conclusion

1 'The VERY odd couple: Shortest man ever (21.5in) meets tallest living person (8ft 1in) outside the Houses of Parliament for Guinness World Record Day', by Stephanie Linning for the MailOnline, 13 November 2014.
2 See esp. Wace, *Grotesques* and Maloney (1976: 37).
3 Suetonius, *Domitianus* 23.2.

Bibliography

Aboutaam, A. and H. Yubero (2007), *Exotics of the Classical World*, Geneva: Phoenix Ancient Art S.A.

Adams, R. (2001), *Sideshow USA. Freaks and the American Cultural Imagination*, Chicago: University of Chicago Press.

Ajootian, A. (1988), '*Ex utroque sexu*: the sleeping hermaphrodite and the myth of Agdistis', *American Journal of Archaeology*, 92: 275–6.

Ajootian, A. (1990), 'Hermaphroditos', *Lexicon Iconographicum Mythologiae Classicae*, V.1: 268–85.

Ajootian, A. (1995), '*Monstrum* or *daimon*: hermaphrodites in ancient art and culture', in B. Berggreen and N. Marinatos (eds), *Greece and Gender*, Bergen: Norwegian Institute at Athens.

Ajootian, A. (1997), 'The only happy couple: hermaphrodites and gender', in A. Koloski-Ostrow and C. Lyons (eds), *Naked Truths. Women, Sexuality and Gender in Classical Art and Archaeology*, London: Routledge.

Allison, P. M. (2004), *Pompeian Households: An Analysis of the Material Culture*, Los Angeles: Cotsen Institute of Archaeology at University of California, Los Angeles.

Ashmole, B. (1929), *A Catalogue of Ancient Marbles at Ince Blundell Hall*, Oxford: Clarendon Press.

Atherton, C. (2000), *Monsters and Monstrosity in Greek and Roman Culture*, Bari: Levante.

Bableon, E. and A. Blanchet (1895), *Catalogue des bronzes antiques de la Bibliothèque nationale*, Paris: E. Leroux.

Bâemont, C., M. Rouvier-Jeanlin and C. Lahanier (1993), 'Les Figurines en Terre cuite gallo-romaines', *Documents d'archâeologie française*, 38.

Baird, L. (1981–83), 'Priapus *Gallinaceus*: the role of the cock in fertility and eroticism in classical antiquity and the middle ages', *Studies in Iconography*, 7–9: 81–111.

Baker, H. S. (1966), *Furniture in the Ancient World: Origins and Evolution, 3100–475 B.C.*, London: The Connoisseur.

Bakhtin, M. (1984), *Rabelais and His World*, trans. H. Iswolsky, Bloomington, Ind.: Indiana University Press.

Barasch, F. K. (1971), *The Grotesque: A Study in Meanings*, The Hague: Mouton.

Baratte, F. (1986), *Le trésor d'orfèvrerie romaine de Boscoréale*, Paris: Editions de la Réunion des musées nationaux.

Barnes, C., M. Oliver and L. Barton (2002), *Disability Studies Today*, Cambridge: Polity Press in association with Blackwell Publishers.

Barnett, R. D. (1982), *Ancient Ivories in the Middle East*, Jerusalem: Institute of Archaeology, Hebrew University of Jerusalem.

Bartman, E. (2002), 'Eros's Flame: Images of Sexy Boys in Roman Ideal Sculpture', *Memoirs of the American Academy in Rome*, Supplementary Volumes 1: 249–79.

Bartman, E. (1992), *Ancient Sculptural Copies in Miniature*, Leiden: E.J. Brill.

Barton, C. (1993), *The Sorrows of the Ancient Romans. The Gladiator and the Monster*, Princeton: Princeton University Press.

Beard, M. and J. Henderson (2001), *Classical Art. From Greece to Rome*, Oxford: Oxford University Press.

Beardsley, G. (1929), *The Negro in Greek and Roman Civilization*, Baltimore: Johns Hopkins Press.

Bernoulli, J. J. (1901), *Griechische Ikonographie mit Ausschluss Alexanders und der Diadochen*, Munich: Hildesheim G. Olms Verlagsbuchhandlung.

Besques, S. (1971–2), *Catalogue raisonné des figurines et reliefs en terre-cuite grecs, étrusques et romains*, Paris: Éditions des Musées nationaux.

Besques, S. (1994), *Figurines et reliefs grecs en terre cuite*, Paris: Réunion des Musées nationaux.

Bieber, M. (1939a), *The History of the Greek and Roman Theatre*, Princeton: Princeton University Press.

Bieber, M. (1939b), 'Mima Saltatricula,' *American Journal of Archaeology*, 43: 640–4.

Bieber, M. (1961), *The Sculpture of the Hellenistic Age*, New York: Columbia University Press.

Bieber, M. (1977), *Ancient Copies: Contributions to the History of Greek and Roman Art*, New York: New York University Press.

Biers, W. (1996), *The Archaeology of Greece*, 2nd edition, Ithaca: Cornell University Press.

Binsfeld, W. (1956), 'Grylloi: ein Beitrag zur Geschichte der antiken Karrikatur', PhD thesis, University of Cologne.

Bissing, V. W. (1903), 'Die Griechisch-Römischen Altertümer im Museum zu Kairo,' *Archaölogischer Anzeiger*, 3: 148–9.

Bloch, R. (1963), *Les prodiges dans l'antiquité classique*, Paris: Presses universitaires de France.

Bode, W. and J. D. Daper (1980), *The Italian Bronze Statuettes of the Renaissance*, New York: H. Grevel & Co.

Bodel, J. (1989), 'Trimalchio and the candelabrum', *Classical Philology*, 84.3: 224–31.

Boehringer, E. and D. Pinkwart (1967), 'Ausgrabung Pergamon', *TürkArkDerg*, 16: 61–5.

Bogden, R. (1988), *Freak Show. Presenting Human Oddities for Amusement and Profit*, Chicago: University of Chicago Press.

Bol, R. (1989), 'Porträt eines Buckligen,' in P.C. Bol (ed.), *Forschungen zur Villa Albani. Katalog der antiken Bildwerke* I, Berlin: G. Mann.

Bonneau, D. (1989), 'L'apotropaïque *abaskantos* en Égypte,' *Revue de l'histoire des religions*, 199: 23–36.

Bonner, C. (1950), *Studies in Magical Amulets, Cheifly Graeco-Egyptian*, Ann Arbor: University of Michigan Press.

Boucher, S. (1970), *Bronzes grecs, hellénistiques, et étrusques (sardes, ibériques,et celtiques), des Musées de Lyon*, Lyon: en dépôt aux Éditions de Boccard, Paris.

Boucher, S. (1973), *Bronzes romains figurés du Musée des beaux-arts de Lyon*, Lyon: en dépôt aux Éditions de Boccard, Paris.

Bouchier, E. S. (1921), *A Short History of Antioch: 300 B.C.– A.D. 1268*, Oxford: Blackwell.

Boyce, A. A. (1937), 'The expiatory rites of 207 B.C.,' *Transactions and Proceedings of the American Philological Association*, 68: 157–71.

Bradley, K. R. (1984), *Slaves and Masters in the Roman Empire. A Study in Social Control*, Oxford: Oxford University Press.

Bradley, M. (2009a), *Colour and Meaning in Ancient Rome*, Cambridge: Cambridge University Press.

Bradley, M. (2009b), 'The Importance of Colour on Ancient Marble Sculpture', *Art History*, 32: 427–57.

Bradley, M. (2011), 'Obesity, corpulence and emaciation in Roman art', *Papers of the British School at Rome*, 79: 1–41.

Braund, S. M. and B. K. Gold (1998), 'Vile Bodies', *Arethusa*, 31.3.

Breccia, E. (1930), *Terrecotte Figurate Greco-Egizie del Museo di Alessandria* II, Bergamo: Officine dell'Istituto italiano d'arti grafiche.

Bregman, J. (1982), *Synesius of Cyrene: Philosopher-Bishop*, Berkeley: University of California Press.

Bremmer, J. (1991), 'Walking, standing and sitting in ancient Greek culture,' in J. Bremmer and H. Roodenburg (eds), *A Cultural History of Gesture: from Antiquity to the Present Day*, Cambridge: Polity Press.

Brendel, O. J. (1953), 'Prolegomena to a book on Roman art,' *Memoirs of the American Academy at Rome*, 21: 7–73.

Brinkmann, V. (1996), 'Farbigkeit der Terrakotten', in F. W. Hamdorf (ed.), *Hauch des Prometheus. Meisterwerke in Ton. Ausst.-Kat. München*, Munich: Staatliche Antikensammlungen und Glyptothek.

Brinkmann, V. and R. Wünsche (2004), *Bunte Götter: die Farbigkeit antiker Skulptur, Ausst. Kat. München*, Munich: Staatliche Antikensammlungen und Glyptothek.

Brisson, L. (2002), *Sexual Ambivalence. Androgyny and Hermaphroditism in Graeco-Roman Antiquity*, trans. J. Lloyd, Berkeley: University of California Press.

Brödner, E. (1951), *Untersuchungen an den Caracallathermen*, Berlin: W. de Gruyter.

Brunet, S. (2003), 'Dwarf athletes in the Roman empire', *Ancient History Bulletin*, 17: 17–32.

Brunet, S. (2004), 'Female and dwarf gladiators', *Mouseion*, 3.4: 145–70.

Buccellato, A., S. Musco, P. Catalano, C. Caldarini, W. Pantano, C. Torri and F. Zabotti (2008), 'Le nécropole de Collatina', in P. Catalano, J. Scheid and S. Verger (eds), *Rome et ses morts. Les Dossiers d'archéologie 330*, Dijon: SFBD Archeologia.

Burford, A. (1972), *Craftsmen in Greek and Roman Society*, Ithaca: Thames and Hudson.

Cadoux, C. (1938), *Ancient Smyrna: A History of the City from the Earliest Times to 324 A.D.*, Oxford: Blackwell.

Cairns, D., ed. (2005), *Body Language in the Greek and Roman Worlds*, Swansea: Classical Press of Wales; Oakville, CT: D. Brown Book Co.

Calandra, E. (1996), *Oltre la Grecia: alle origini del filellenismo di Adriano*, Naples: Edizioni scientifiche italiane.

Calza, G. (1939), 'Die Taverne der Sieben Weisen in Ostia', *Die Antike*, 15: 99–115.

Canci, A., L. Nencioni, S. Minozzi, P. Catalano, D. Caramella and G. Fornaciari (2005), 'A case of healing spinal infection from Classical Rome', *International Journal of Osteoarchaeology*, 15: 77–83.

Capasso, L. (1999), 'Brucellosis at Herculaneum (79AD)', *International Journal of Osteoarchaeology*, 9: 277–88.

Capelle, W. (1953), 'Zwei Quellen des Heliodor', *Rheinisches Museum für Philologie*, 96: 175–80.

Carelli, F. (1755–1831), *Le antichita di Ercolano esposte*, Naples: Regia stamperia.

Carpenter, T. (1986), *Dionysian Imagery in Archaic Greek Art: Its Development in Black-Figure Vase Painting*, Oxford: Clarendon Press.

Carpino, A. (2003), *Discs of Splendor: The Relief Mirrors of the Etruscans*, Wisconsin: University of Wisconsin Press.

Carpino, A. (2008), 'Reflections from the Tomb: Mirrors as Grave Goods in Late Classical and Hellenistic Tarquinia', *Journal of the Etruscan Foundation*, 11: 1–33.

Casson, L. (1974), *Travel in the Ancient World*, Baltimore: Johns Hopkins University Press.

Catalano, P., S. Minozzi and W. Pantano (2001), 'Le necropolis romane di età imperial: Un contributo all'interpretazione del popolamento e della qualità della vita nell'antica Roma', in L. Quilici and S. Quilici Gigli (eds), *Atlante tematico di topografia antica* 10. Rome: L'Erma di Bretschneider.

Catherine, A., ed. (1998), *Monsters and Monstrosity in Greek and Roman Culture*, Bari: Levante.

Cèbe, J-P. (1966), *La caricature et la parodie dans le monde romain antique*, Paris: E. de Boccard.

Charbonneaux, J. (1936), *Les terres-cuites grecques*, Paris: L. Reynaud.

Charbonneaux, J. (1962), *Greek Bronzes*, trans. K. Watson, London: Elek Books.

Charcot, J. M. and P. Richer (1972), *Les difformes et les malades dans l'Art*, Amsterdam: B.M. Israël.

Charlier, P. (2008), 'Ce que la paléo-pathologie révèle du sort des individus mal formés dans l'Antiquité gréco-romaine', *La Revue du Praticien*, 54: 921–5.

Chesterman, J. (1974), *Classical Terracotta Figures*, London: Ward Lock.

Cimok, F. (2000), *Antioch Mosaics: A Corpus*, Istanbul: A Turizm Yayinlari.

Clarke, J. (1996), 'Hypersexual black men in Augustan baths: ideal somatotypes and apotropaic magic', in N. Kampen (ed.), *Sexuality in Ancient Art: Near East, Egypt, Greece, and Italy*, Cambridge: Cambridge University Press.

Clarke, J. (1998), *Looking at Lovemaking: Constructions of Sexuality in Roman Art, 100 B.C.–A.D. 250.*, Berkeley: University of California Press.

Clarke, J. (2002), 'Look who's laughing at sex', in D. Fredrick (ed.), *The Roman Gaze. Vision, Power, and the Body*, Baltimore: Johns Hopkins University Press.

Clarke, J. (2003), *Art in the Lives of Ordinary Romans*, Berkeley: University of California Press.

Clarke, J. (2007a), 'Three uses of the pygmy and the Aethiops at Pompeii', in L. Bricault, M. J. Versluys and P. Meyboom (eds), *Nile into Tiber. Egypt in the Roman World*, Leiden: Brill.

Clarke, J. (2007b), *Looking at Laughter: Humor, Power and Transgression in Roman Visual Culture, 100 B.C.–A.D. 250*. Berkeley: University of California Press.

Cocke, R. (1980), 'Masaccio and the Spinario, Piero and the *pothos*: Observations on the reception of the antique in Renaissance painting', *Zeitschrift für Kunstgeschichte*, 43.1: 21–32.

Cohen, B., ed. (2000), *Not the Classical Ideal: Athens and the Construction of the Other in Greek Art*, Leiden: Brill.

Cohen, C. (2003), *La Femme des origines: Images de la femme dans la préhistoire occidentale*, Paris: Belin-Herscher.

Cohon, R. (1984), 'Greek and Roman Stone Table Supports with Decorated Reliefs', PhD thesis, New York University.

Cokayne, K. (2003), *Experiencing Old Age in Ancient Rome*, London: Routledge.

Comstock, M. and C. Vermeule (1971), *Greek, Etruscan, & Roman Bronzes in the Museum of Fine Arts, Boston*. Boston: Museum of Fine Arts.

Comstock, M. and C. Vermeule (1988), *Sculpture in Stone and Bronze: Additions to the Collections of Greek, Etruscan, and Roman Art, 1971–1988, in the Museum of Fine Arts, Boston*, Boston: Museum of Fine Arts.

Cooney, J. D. (1966), 'On the meaning of bj3.w', *Zeitschrift für ägyptische Sprache und Altertumskunde*, 93: 43–7.

Corbeill, A. (1996), *Controlling Laughter. Political Humor in the Late Roman Republic*, Princeton: Princeton University Press.

Corker, M. and T. Shakespeare (2002), *Disability/Postmodernity: Embodying Disability Theory*, London: Continuum.

Croom, A. T. (2007), *Roman Furniture*, Stroud: Tempus.

Cruse, A. (2004), *Roman Medicine*, Stroud: Tempus.

Dacos, N. (1969), *La Découverte de la Domus Aurea et la Formation des Grotesques à la Renaissance*, London: Warburg Institute.

D'Arms, J. H. (1991), 'Slaves at Roman *convivia*', in W. J. Slater (ed.), *Dining in a Classical Context*, Ann Arbor: University of Michigan Press.

Dasen, V. (1993), *Dwarfs in Ancient Egypt and Greece*, Oxford: Oxford University Press.

Dasen, V. (1994), 'Pygmaioi', *Lexicon Iconographicum Mythologiae Classicae*, VII.1: 594–601.

Dasen, V. (2006), 'L'enfant qui ne grandit pas', *Medicina nei secoli*, 18.2: 1–13.

Dasen, V. (2013), 'Des musiciens différents? Nains danseurs et musiciens dans le monde hellénistique et romain', in S. Emerit (ed.), *Le statut du musician dans la Méditerranée ancienne: Égypte, Mésopotamie, Grèce et Rome*, Cairo: Institut Français d'Archéologie Orientale.

Davies, P. V. (1969), *Macrobius: The Saturnalia*, New York: Columbia University Press.

Dawson, W. R. (1927), 'Pygmies, dwarfs and hunchbacks in ancient Egypt', *Annals of Medical History*, 9/4: 315–26.

DeLaine, J. (1997), *The Baths of Caracalla: A Study in the Design, Construction, and Ecomonics of Large Scale Building Projects in Rome*, Rhode Island: Journal of Roman Archaeology.

Delatte, A. (1954), 'Une clochette magique antique', *Bulletin de la Classe de l'Académie royale de Belgique, 5e ser.*, 40: 254–76.

Delcourt, M. (1961), *Hermaphrodite: mythes et rites de la bisexualité dans l'antiquité classique*, Paris: Presses Universitaires de France.

Delivorrias, A., G. Berger-Doer and A. Kossarz-Deissmann (1984), *Aphrodite, Lexicon Inconographicom Mythologiae Classicae*, II. I: 85–6.

Dessau, H. (1892–1916), *Inscriptiones Latinae Selectae*, 3 vols, Berlin: Apud Weidmannos.

DeVillefosse, A. (1899), 'Le trésor de Boscoréale', *Mon. Piot*, 5: 1–290.

Devisse, J. (1979), *The Image of the Black in Western Art*, trans. by W. G. Ryan, New York: William Morrow.

DeVos, M. (1933), 'Camillo Paderni, la tradizione antiquarian romana e I collezionisti inglesi', *Ercolano*, 1738–1988.

Dickie, M.W. (1993), 'Βασκάνια, προβασκάνια and προσβασκάνια', *Glotta*, 71: 174–7.

Dickie, M. W. (1995), 'A joke in old comedy: Aristophanes fragment 607PCG', *Classical Philology*, 90: 241–5.

Dieterich, A. (1897), *Pucinella: Pompejanische Wandbilder und römische Satyrspiele*, Leipzig: B.G. Teubner.

Dingwall, E. J. (1925), *Male Infibulation*, London: John Bale, sons & Danielsson, Ltd.

Di Nola, A. (1974), 'Riso ed oscenita', in *Antropologia religiosa: introduzione al problema e campioni di ricerca*, Florence: Vallecchi.

Dover, K. J. (1978), *Greek Homosexuality*, London: Duckworth.

DuBois, P. (2003), *Slaves and Other Objects*, Chicago: University of Chicago Press.

Dulaure, J. A. (1890), *Priapic Divinities and Phallic Rites*, Paris: I. Liseux.

Du Mersan, M. (1838), *Histoire du cabinet des médailles, antiques et pierres gravées*, Paris: M. Du Mersan.

Dunbabin, K. (1986), 'Sic erimus cuncti. The skeleton in Graeco-Roman art', *Jahrbuch des Deutschen Archäologischen Instituts*, 101: 185–255.

Dunbabin, K. (1989), '*Baiarum grata voluptas*: pleasures and dangers of the baths', *Papers of the British School at Rome*, 57: 6–49.

Dunbabin, K. (1994) 'Review of Dasen's *Dwarfs in Ancient Egypt and Greece*', *Bryn Mawr Classical Review*, 94.09.07, http://bmcr.brynmawr.edu/1994/94.09.07.html (accessed 2 February 2015).

Dunbabin, K. (2003), *The Roman Banquet: Images of Conviviality*, Cambridge: Cambridge University Press.

Dunbabin, K. and M. W. Dickie (1983), '*Invida Rumpantur Pectora*. The iconography of *phthonos/invidia* in Graeco-Roman art', *Jahrbuch für Antike und Christentum*, 26: 7–37.

Dundes, A. (1981), *The Evil Eye: A Folklore Casebook*, New York: Garland Publishing.

Dwyer, E. (1982), *Pompeian Domestic Sculpture: A Study of Five Pompeian Houses and their Contents*, Rome: G. Bretschneider.

Edgar, C. C. and C. Cowan (1903), *Catalogue Général des Antiquités Égyptiennes du Musée du Caire*, Cairo: Institut Français d'Archéologie Orientale.

Edwards, C. (1993), *The Politics of Immorality in Ancient Rome*, Cambridge: Cambridge University Press.

Edwards, C. (1997), 'Unspeakable professions, public performance and prostitution in Ancient Rome,' in J. Hallett and M. B. Skinner (eds), *Roman Sexualities*, Princeton: Princeton University Press.

Edwards, C. (2005), 'Archetypally Roman? Representing Seneca's ageing body', in A. Hopkins and M. Wyke (eds), *Roman Bodies: Antiquity to the Eighteenth Century*, London: British School at Rome.

Eichler, F. (1951), 'Review of Dorothy Hill Kent. Catalogue of classical bronze sculpture in the Walters Art Gallery', *Gnomon*, 23: 59–61.

Elderkin, W. (1934), *Antioch on-the-Orontes: 1, The Excavations of 1932*, Princeton: Pub. for the Committee by the Department of Art and Archeology of Princeton University.

Elworthy, F. T. (1895), *The Evil Eye: An Account of this Ancient and Widespread Superstition*, London: Murray.

Emmanuel, M. (1916), *The Antique Greek Dance: After Sculptured and Painted Figures*, trans. by H. J. Beauley, New York: John Lane.

Eschebach, H. (1979), *Die Stabianer Thermen in Pomeji*, Berlin: de Gruyter.

Essen, C. C. van (1933), *Historische Opmerkingen over de statuetten uit Tanagra*, Amsterdam: Koninklijk Nederlands Instituut Rome.

Evans, E. (1969), 'Physiognomics in the ancient world', *Transactions and Proceedings of the American Philological Association*, 59.5: 5–101.

Fagan, G. (1999), *Bathing in Public in the Roman World*, Ann Arbor: University of Michigan Press.

Falkner, M. and M. de Luce (1989), *Old Age in Greek and Latin Literature*, Albany: State University of New York Press.

Fantham, E. (1994), *Women in the Classical World: Image and Text*, New York: Oxford University Press.

Faraone, C. (1992), *Talismans and Trojan Horses. Talismanic Statues in Greek Myth and Ritual*, Oxford: Oxford University Press.

Ferris, I. M. (2000), *Enemies of Rome: Barbarians through Roman Eyes*, Stroud: Sutton.

Fiedler, L. (1978), *Freaks: Myths and Images of the Secret Self*, New York: Simon and Schuster.

Fischer, J. (1998), 'Der Zwerg, der Phallos und der Buckel', *Chronique d'Egypte*, 73: 327–61.

Fischer, J. and T. Zachmann (1994), *Griechisch-römische Terrakotten aus Ägypten: Die Sammlungen Sieglin und Schreiber: Dresden, Leipzig, Stuttgart, Tübingen*, Tübingen: E. Wasmuth.

Fitton, J. L. (1992), *Ivory in Greece and the Eastern Mediterranean from the Bronze Age to the Hellenistic Period*, London: Dept. of Greek and Roman Antiquities, British Museum.

Flower, H. (1996), *Ancestor Masks and Aristocratic Power in Roman Culture*, Oxford: Clarendon Press.

Foerster, R. (1893), *Scriptores Physiognomonici Graeci et Latini*, Lipsiae: B. G. Teubneri.

Fowler, H. B. (1989), *The Hellenistic Aesthetic*, Madison: University of Wisconsin Press.

Foxhall, L. and J. Salmon, eds (1998), *When Men were Men: Masculinity, Power and Identity in Classical Antiquity*, London: Routledge.

Fredrick, D. (2002), *The Roman Gaze: Vision, Power and the Body*, Baltimore: Johns Hopkins University Press.

Friedländer, L. (1913), *Roman Life and Manners under the Early Empire*, trans. L. Magnus, London: G. Routledge.

Froehner, W. (1873), *Les musées de France: recueil de monuments antiques*, Paris: J. Rothschild.

Froehner, W. (1886), *Collection H. Hoffmann: catalogue des objets d'art antiques, terres cuites, bijoux, verrerie*, Paris: Hôtel Drouot.

Fuchs, W. (1963), *Der Schiffsfund von Mahdia*, Tübingen: F. Wasmuth.

Furtwängler, A. and P. Wolters (1910), *Beschreibung der Glyptothek König Ludwigs I zu München*, Munich: Ackermann.

Garland, R. (1995, 2010), *The Eye of the Beholder. Deformity and Disability in the Graeco-Roman World*, London: Bristol Classical Press.

Garmaise, M. (1996), 'Studies in the Representation of Dwarfs in Hellenistic and Roman Art', PhD thesis, McMaster University.

Gasparri, C. (1983/4), 'Sculture proveniente dale Terme di Caracalla e di Diocleziano', *RivIstArch*, Supplement III.6–7: 133–50.

Gassowska, B. (1966), '*Cirrus in vertice* – one of the problems in Roman athlete iconography', in M. L. Bernhard (ed.), *Mélanges offerts à Kazimierz Michalowski*, Warsaw: Państwowe Wydawn. Naukowe.

Gauckler, P. (1895), *Musées d'Algérie de la Tunisie 4, Musée de Cherchel*, Paris: E. Leroux.

Gazda, E. (1991), *Roman Art in the Private Sphere: New Perspectives on the Architecture and Decor of the Domus, Villa, and Insula*, Ann Arbor: University of Michigan Press.

Gazda, E. (2002), *The Ancient Art of Emulation: Studies in Artistic Originality and Tradition from the Present to Classical Antiquity*, Ann Arbor: University of Michigan Press.

Gerhard, E. (1965), *Etruskischer Spiegel*, vol. IV, Rome: Ardita.

Gerhard, E., K. O. Müller, T. Panofka, O. von Stackelberg and F. G. Welcker (1833), *Hyperboreisch-römische Studien für Archäologie*, Berlin: Duncker und Humblot.

Germain, S. (1969), *Les mosaïques de Timgad: étude descriptive et analytique*, Paris: Éditions du Centre national de la recherche scientifique.

Girardon, C. F. (1993), 'Ancient Medicine and Anatomical Votives in Italy', *Bulletin of the Institute of Archaeology*, 30: 29–40.

Giuliani, L. (1987), 'Die seligen Krüppel. Zur Deutung von Mißgestalten in der hellenistischen Kleinkunst', *Archaölogischer Anzeiger*, 102: 701–21.

Giuliani, L. (1989), 'Bildnis-Statuette des Diogenes', in P. C. Bol (ed.), *Forschungen zur Villa Albani. Katalog der antiken Bildwerke* I, Berlin: G. Mann.

Giuliano, A. (1953), 'La Afrodite Callipige di Siracusa', *Archeologia Classica*, 5: 210–14.

Gleason, M. (1995), *Making Men. Sophists and Self-Representation in Ancient Rome*, Princeton: Princeton University Press.

Goddard, J. (1994), 'The tyrant at table', in J. Elsner and J. Masters (eds), *Reflections of Nero: Culture, History, & Representation*, Chapel Hill: University of North Carolina Press.

Goldhill, S. (2002), *Who Needs Greek? Contests in the Cultural History of Hellenism*, Cambridge: Cambridge University Press.

Goldman, H. (1943), 'Two terracotta figurines from Tarsus', *American Journal of Archaeology*, 47: 22–34.

Gould, J. (1973), '*Hiketeia*', *Journal of Hellenic Studies*, 93: 74–103.

Gourevitch, D. (1985), 'L'obésité et son traitement dans le monde romain', *History and Philosophy of the Life Sciences*, 7: 195–215.

Gowers, E. (1993), *The Loaded Table: Representations of Food in Roman Literature*, Oxford: Clarendon Press.

Graf, F. (1991), 'The gestures of Roman actors and orators', in J. Bremmer and H. Roodenburg (eds), *A Cultural History of Gesture: from Antiquity to the Present Day*, Cambridge: Polity Press.

Graham, E-J. (2013), 'Disparate lives or disparate deaths? Post-mortem treatment of the body and the articulation of difference', in C. Laes, C. F. Goodey and M. L. Rose (eds), *Disabilities in Roman Antiquity: Disparate Bodies A Capite ad Calcem*, Leiden: Brill.

Grimm, G. (1969), *Die Zeugnisse ägyptischer Religion und Kunstelemente im römischen Deutschland*, Leiden: E.J. Brill.

Grmek, M. (1988), 'Les affections de la colonne vertébrale dans l'iconographie médicale et les arts antiques', *Histoire et Archeologie*, 123: 52–61.

Grmek, M. (1989), *Diseases in the Ancient Greek World*, trans. by M. Muellner and L. Muellner, Baltimore: Johns Hopkins University Press.

Grmek, M. and D. Gourevitch (1987), 'L'obésité et ses représentations figurées dans l'Antiquité', *Archeologie et Medecine*, VII: 355–67.

Grmek, M. and D. Gourevitch (1998), *Les Maladies dans l'art Antique*, Paris: Fayard.

Gros, R. (1987), 'Les thermes dans la Rome antique', *Histoires des Sciences Médicales*, 21: 45–50.

Gruen, E. (1992), *Culture and National Identity in Republican Rome*, Ithaca: Cornell University Press.

Grummond, N. de (1982), 'The usage of etruscan mirrors', in N. T. de Grummond (ed.), *A Guide to Etruscan Mirrors*, Tallahassee: Archaeological News.

Grummond, N. de (1991), 'Etruscan twins and mirror images: the Dioskouroi at the door', *Yale Bulletin*, 10: 10–31.

Gunderson, E. (2000), *Staging Masculinity. The Rhetoric of Performance in the Roman World*, Ann Arbor: University of Michigan Press.

Hackmann, O. (1904), 'Die Polyphemsage in der Volksüberlieferung', PhD thesis, Helsingors Universitet.

Haj, F. (1970), *Disability in Antiquity*, New York: Philosophical Library.

Hall, E. (1989), *Inventing the Barbarian: Greek Self-definition through Tragedy*, Oxford: Clarendon Press.

Hall, E. (1998), 'Ithyphallic males behaving badly; or the gender dynamics of satyr drama', in M. Wyke (ed.), *Parchments of Gender: Reading the Bodies of Antiquity*, Oxford: Clarendon Press.

Hallett, C. (2005), *The Roman Nude: Heroic Portrait Statuary 200 BC–AD 300*, Oxford: Oxford University Press.

Halperin, D. (1990), *One Hundred Years of Greek Homosexuality*, New York: Routledge.

Harpham, G. (1982), *On the Grotesque: Strategies of Contradiction in Art and Literature*, Princeton: Princeton University Press.

Hartmann, R. (1912), 'Ein Phallobates,' *Archaölogischer Anzeiger*, 27: 13–16.

Hartog, F. (1988), *The Mirror of Herodotus: The Representation of the Other in the Writing of History*, trans. by J. Lloyd, Berkeley: University of California Press.

Haskell, F. and N. Penny (1981), *Taste and the Antique: The Lure of Classical Sculpture, 1500–1900*, New Haven: Yale University Press.

Hatt, J-J. (1954), 'Les fouilles de Strasbourg en 1953 et 1954. Découverte d'un dépotoir de céramique', *Gallia*, 12.1: 323–44.

Havelock, C. M. (1971), *Hellenistic Art: The Art of the Classical World from the Death of Alexander the Great to the Battle of Actium*, Greenwich: New York Graphic Society.

Haynes, D. (1992), *The Technique of Greek Bronze Statuary*, Mainz: P. von Zabern.

Hekster, O. (2002), *Commodus: An Emperor at the Crossroads*, Amsterdam: J.C. Gieben.

Helbig, W. (1868), *Wandgemälde der vom Vesuv verschütteten Städte Campaniens*, Leipzig: Breitkopf und Härtel.

Helbig, W. (1963–72), *Führer durch die öffentlichen Sammlungen klassischer Altertümer in Rom*, Tübingen: E. Wasmuth.

Hercher, R. (1965), *Epistolographi graeci*, Amsterdam: A. M. Hakkert.

Herter, H. (1932), *De Priapo*, Giessen: Alfred Töpelmann.

Hesberg, H. von (1988), 'Bildsyntax und Erzählweise in der hellenistischen Flächenkunst', *Jahrbuch des Deutschen Archäologischen Instituts*, 103: 309–65.

Heuzey, L. (1923), *Catalogue des figurines antiques de terre cuite: figurines orientales et figurines des îles asiatiques*, Paris: Musées nationaux.

Higgins, R. A. (1967), *Greek Terracottas*, London: Methuen.

Hill, D. K. (1949), *Catalogue of Classical Bronze Sculpture in the Walters Art Gallery*, Baltimore: Walters Art Gallery.

Himmelman, N. (1971), *Archäologisches zum Problem der griechischen Sklaverei*, Mainz: Verlag der Akademie der Wissenschaften und der Literatur.

Himmelman, N. (1981), 'Realistic art in Alexandria', *Proceedings of the British Academy*, 67: 193–207.

Himmelman, N. (1983), *Alexandria und der Realismus in der griechischen Kunst*, Tübingen: E. Wasmuth.

Hoffmann, H. (1960), 'Neuerwerbungen Hamburg', *Archaölogischer Anzeiger*, 75: 120–22.

Holländer, E. (1912), *Plastik und Medizin*, Stuttgart: F. Enke.

Hopkins, A. and M. Wyke, eds (2005), *Roman Bodies: Antiquity to the Eighteenth Century*, London: British School at Rome.

Hopkins, K. (1978), *Conquerors and Slaves*, Cambridge: Cambridge University Press.

Hopkins, K. (1993), 'New evidence for Roman slavery', *Past and Present*, 138: 3–27.

Hughes, A. and E. Ranfft, eds (1997), *Sculpture and its Reproductions*, London: Reaktion Books.

Jahn, O. (1843), *Archäologische Beiträge*, Berlin.

Jahn, O. (1846), *Die hellenische Kunst*, Greifswald.

Jahn, O. (1855), *Über den Aberglauben des bösen Blicks bei den Alten*, Leipzig.

Jahn, O. (1857), *Die Wandgemälde des Columbariums in der Villa Pamfili*, Munich: Verlag der k. Academie.

Jantzen, U. (1958), 'Statuette eines Buckligen', *Jahrbuch der Hamburger Kunstsammlungen*, Band 3: 47–51.

Jashemski, W. F. (1987), *The Gardens of Pompeii: Herculaneum and the Villas Destroyed by Vesuvius*, New York: Caratzas.

Jashemski, W. F. and E. B. Macdougall, eds (1981), *Ancient Roman Gardens*, Washington: Dumbarton Oaks Trustees for Harvard University.

Jedrkiewicz, S. (1989), *Sapere e paradosso nell'antichità: Esopo e la favola*, Rome: Edizioni dell'Ateneo.

Johansen, F. (1995), *Catalogue of Roman Portraits, Ny Carlsberg Glyptotek*, trans. by D. A. Marmorstein, Copenhagen: Ny Carlsberg glyptotek.

Johns, C. (1982), *Sex or Symbol: Erotic Images of Greece and Rome*, London: British Museum Publications.

Kampen, N. (1996), *Sexuality in Ancient Art: Near East, Egypt, Greece, and Italy*, Cambridge: Cambridge University Press.

Kapossy, B. (1969), *Brunnenfiguren der hellenistischen und römischen Zeit*, Zurich: Juris Druck & Verlag.

Kayser, W. J. (1981), *The Grotesque in Art and Literature*, trans. U. Weisstein, New York: Columbia University Press.

Keith-Bennet, J. and L. Grierson (1980), *An Introduction to Ancient Art at the Wadworth Atheneum, Hartford, Connecticut*, Hartford, CT: Wadsworth Atheneum.

Kenseth, J. (1998), 'The virtue of littleness: small-scale sculptures of the Italian renaissance', in S. B. McHam (ed.), *Looking at Italian Rennaisance Sculpture*, Cambridge: Cambridge University Press.

Keuls, E. (1993), *The Reign of the Phallus: Sexual Politics in Ancient Athens*, Berkeley: University of California Press.

Kilmer, M. F. (1997), 'Painters and pederasts: ancient art, sexuality, and social history', in M. Golden and P. Toohey (eds), *Inventing Ancient Culture. Historicism, Periodization and the Ancient World*, London: Routledge.

Kleiner, D. (1992), *Roman Sculpture*, New Haven: Yale University Press.

Knight, R. P. (1974), *A Discourse on the Worship of Priapus*, Secaucus: University Books.

Kondoleon, C. (2000), *Antioch: The Lost Ancient City*, Princeton: Princeton University Press.

Kozloff, A. and D. Mitten (1988), *The Gods Delight: The Human Figure in Classical Bronze*, Cleveland: Cleveland Museum of Art in cooperation with Indiana University Press.

Kraemer, Jr., C. (1931), 'A Greek element in Egyptian dancing', *American Journal of Archaeology*, 35: 125–38.

Krencker, D., L. Hussong and H. Cüppers (1929), *Die Trierer Kaiserthermen*, Augsburg: Filser.

Krzyszkowska, O. (1996), 'Furniture in the Aegean Bronze Age', in G. Herrmann (ed.), *The Furniture of Western Asia, Ancient and Traditional*, Mainz: Philipp von Zabern.

Kudlien, F. and R. Durling (1991), *Galen's Method of Healing: Proceedings of the 1982 Galen Symposium*, Leiden: Brill.

Kunz, J. and I. Nippert (1986), *Genetics and Malformations in Art*, Berlin: Grosse Verlag.

Kunzl, E. (2002), *Souvenirs und Devotionalien*, Mainz am Rhein: P. von Zabern.

Laes, C. (2008), 'Learning from silence: disabled children in Roman antiquity', *Arctos*, 42: 85–122.

Laes, C. (2011), 'Silent witnesses: deaf-mutes in Graeco-Roman antiquity', *Classical World*, 104.4: 451–73.

Laes, C. (2013), 'Silent history? Speech impairment in Roman antiquity', in C. Laes, C. F. Goodey and M. L. Rose (eds), *Disabilities in Roman Antiquity: Disparate Bodies A Capite ad Calcem*, Leiden: Brill.

Lamb, W. (1929), *Greek and Roman Bronzes*, London: Metheun.

Lanciani, R. (1888), *Ancient Rome in the Light of Recent Discoveries*, Boston: Houghton Mifflin.

Lanciani, R. (1897), *The Ruins and Excavations of Ancient Rome*, New York: Blom.

Lapatin, K. (2001), *Chryselephantine Statuary in the Ancient Mediterranean World*, Oxford: Oxford University Press.

La Penna (1962), 'Il Romanzo di Esopo', *Athenaeum*, 40: 270–84.

Laubscher, H-P. (1982), *Fischer und Landleute: Studien zur hellenistischen Genreplastik*, Mainz am Rhein: v. Zabern.

Laumonier, A. (1946), 'Terre-cuites d'Asie Mineure', *Bulletin de correspondance hellénique*, 70: 312–18.

Lawler, L. (1964), *The Dance in Ancient Greece*, London: A. & C. Black.

Leppert, R. (2007), *Nude: The Cultural Rethoric of the Body in the Art of Western Modernity*, Boulder: Westview Press.

Levi, D. (1941), 'The evil eye and the lucky hunchback', in R. Stillwell (ed.), *Antioch-on-the-Orontes* 3, Princeton: Committee by the Department of Art and Archeology of Princeton University.

Levi, D. (1947), 'House of the evil eye – lower level', *Antioch Mosaic Pavements*, Princeton: Princeton University Press.

Lewis, C. T. and C. Short, eds (1879), *A Latin Dictionary*, Oxford: Oxford University Press.

Leyenaar-Plaisier, P. G. (1984), 'Smyrne et la culture hellénistique', *Les Dossiers du Musée du Louvre*, 81.2: 69–80.

Lézine, A. (1961), *Architecture romaine d'Afrique: Recherches et mises au point*, Paris: Presses universitaires de France.

Liddell, H. G. and R. Scott (1958), *A Greek–English Lexicon*, 9th edition, Oxford: Oxford University Press.

Liebeschuetz, J. H. W. G. (1972), *Antioch: City and Imperial Administration in the Later Roman Empire*, Oxford: Clarendon Press.

Lippold, G. (1912), *Griechische Porträtstatuen*, Munich: Bruckmann.

Lippold, G. (1923), *Kopien und Umbildungen griechischer Statuen*, Munich: Beck.

Lippold, G. (1937), *Die Sculpturen des Vaticanischen Museums*, Berlin: G. Reimer.

Lissarrague, F. (1990a), 'The sexual life of satyrs', in D. Halperin, J. Winkler and F. I. Zeitlin (eds), *Before Sexuality. The Construction of the Erotic Experience in the Ancient Greek World*, Princeton: Princeton University Press.
Lissarrague, F. (1990b), 'Why satyrs are good to represent', in J. J. Winkler and F. I. Zeitlin (eds), *Nothing to do with Dionysos? Athenian Drama in Its Social Context*, Princeton: Princeton University Press.
Lissarrague, F. (1993), 'On the wildness of satyrs', in T. H. Carpenter and C. A. Faraone (eds), *Masks of Dionysos*, Ithaca: Cornell University Press.
Lissarrague, F. (2000), 'Aesop, between man and beast: ancient portraits and illustrations', in B. Cohen (ed.), *Not the Classical Ideal. Athens and the Construction of the Other in Greek Art*, Leiden: Brill.
Littré, E. (1839–61), *Hippocrates: Oeuvres completes*, Paris: J.B. Baillière.
Liverani, P. and H. Bankel (2004), *I colori del bianco: policromia nella scultura antica*, Rome: De Luca.
Lullies, R. (1962), 'Neuerwerbungen der Antikensammlungen in München, 1958–1961', *Archaölogischer Anzeiger*, 77: 594–631.
MacBain, B. (1982), *Prodigy and Expiation. A Study in Religion and Politics in Republican Rome*, Latomus vol. 177, Brussels: Latomus.
Maiuri, A. (1932), *La casa del Menandro e il suo tesoro di argenteria*, Rome: Libreria dello stato.
Maiuri, A. (1956), *Pompei: i nuovi scavi, la villa dei misteri, l'antiquarium*, Rome: Ist. poligrafico dello Stato, Libreria.
Maloney, C. (1976), *The Evil Eye*, New York: Columbia University Press.
Manderscheid, H. (1981), *Die Skulpturenausstattung der kaiserzeitlichen Thermenanlagen*, Berlin: Mann.
Manderscheid, H. (1988), *Bibliographie zum römischen Badewesen*, Munich: In Kommission bei Wasmuth.
Mansuelli, G. (1958), *Galleria degli Uffizi: le sculture*, Rome: Istituto poligrafico dello Stato, Libreria dello Stato.
Marcadé, J. (1969), *Au musée de Délos, étude sur la sculpture hellénistique en ronde bosse découverte dans l'île*, Paris: Éditions E. de Boccard.
Marvin, M. (1983), 'Free-standing sculptures in the baths of Caracalla', *American Journal of Archaeology*, 87: 347–84.
Marvin, M. (1989), 'Copying in Roman sculpture, the replica series', *Studies in the History of Art*, 20: 29–45.
Masséglia, J. (2012), 'Reasons to be cheerful: conflicting emotions in the Drunken Old Women of Munich and Rome', in A. Chaniotis (ed.), *Unveiling Emotions*, Stuttgart: Franz Steiner Verlag.

Masséglia, J. (2013), 'Feeling low: social status and emotional display in Hellenistic art,' in A. Chaniotis and P. Ducrey (eds), *Unveiling Emotions* II, Stuttgart: Franz Steiner Verlag.

Masséglia, J. (2015), *Body Language in Hellenistic Art and Society*, Oxford: Oxford University Press.

Mattusch, C. C. (1996), *Classical Bronzes: The Art and Craft of Greek and Roman Statuary*, Ithaca: Cornell University Press.

McHardy, F. and E. Marshall (2004), *Women's Influence on Classical Civilization*, London: Routledge.

McKay, M. J. (1985), 'Pygmy Landscapes in Roman Art', PhD thesis, University of Toronto.

McNiven, T. J. (1995), 'The unheroic penis: otherness exposed', *Source: Special Issue: Representations of the Other in Athenian Art*, 15.1: 10–16.

McNiven, T. J. (2000), 'Behaving like an other: telltale gestures in Athenian vase painting,' in B. Cohen (ed.), *Not the Classical Ideal. Athens and the Construction of the Other in Greek Art*, Leiden: Brill.

Meige, H. (1897), 'Le mal de pott dans l'art antique', *Travaux de Neurologie Chirurgicale* II.

Metzler, D. (1971), *Porträt und Gesellschaft: Über die Entstehung des griechischen Porträts in der Klassik*, Münster: D. Metzler.

Meyboom, P. and M. J. Versluys (2005), 'The meaning of dwarfs in Nilotic scenes', in L. Bricault, M. J. Versluys and P. Meyboom (eds), *Nile into Tiber: Egypt in the Roman World*, Leiden: Brill.

Michler, M. (1993), '*Principis Medicus*: Antonius Musa', in H. Temporini (ed.), *Aufstieg und Niedergang der römischen Welt*, 2.37.1. Berlin: de Gruyter.

Mitchell, A. G. (2013), 'Disparate bodies in ancient artefacts: the function of caricature and pathological grotesques among Roman terracotta figurines', in C. Laes, C. F. Goodey and M. L. Rose (eds), *Disabilities in Roman Antiquity: Disparate Bodies A Capite ad Calcem*, Leiden: Brill.

Mitchell, D. and S. Snyder (1997), *The Body and Physical Difference: Discourses of Disability in the Humanities*, Ann Arbor: University of Michigan Press.

Mitten, D. and S. Doeringer (1967), *Master Bronzes from the Classical World*, Mainz on Rhine: P. von Zabern.

Montague, J. (1989), *Roman Baroque Sculpture. The Industry of Art*, New Haven: Yale University Press.

Montseratt, D. (1998), *Changing Bodies, Changing Meanings: Studies on the Human Body in Antiquity*, London: Routledge.

Moon, W. (1995), *Polykleitos, the Doryphoros, and Tradition*, Madison, Wis.: University of Wisconsin Press.

Moore, J. (1781), *A View of Society and Manners in Italy*, London: W. Strahan; and T. Cadell, in the Strand.

Morgan, L. (1997), '*Achilleae Comae*: hair and heroism according to Domitian', *Classical Quarterly*, 47.1: 209–14.

Moss, C. (1988), 'Roman Marble Tables', PhD thesis, Princeton University.

Murray, A. S. (1898), *Greek Bronzes*, London: Seeley.

Naerebout, F. G. (1997), *Attractive Performances. Ancient Greek Dance: Three Preliminary Studies*, Amsterdam: J.C. Gieben.

Nappo, S. (1998), *Pompeii: Guide to the Lost City*, London: Weidenfeld & Nicolson.

Neudecker, R. (1994), *Die Pracht der Latrine*, Munich: Verlag Dr. Friedrich Pfeil.

Neugebauer, K. (1951), *Die griechischen Bronzen der klassischen Zeit und des Hellenismus*, Berlin: Akademie-Verlag.

Nicholson, F. (1968), *Ancient Life in Miniature: An Exhibition of Classical Terracottas from Private Collections in England*, Birmingham: Birmingham Museum & Art Gallery.

Nicole, J. (1906), *Un Catalogue d'oeuvres d'art conservées à Rome à l'époque impériale*, Geneva: W. Kundig & Fils.

Nicoll, A. (1931), *Masks, Mimes and Miracles. Studies in the Popular Theatre*, London: Harrap.

North, H. (1966), *Sophrosyne. Self-knowledge and Self-restraint in Greek Literature*, Ithaca: Cornell University Press.

Ogdens, D. (1997), *The Crooked Kings of Ancient Greece*, London: Duckworth.

Oggiano-Bitar, H. (1984), *Bronzes figurés antiques des Bouches-du-Rhône*, Paris: Éditions du Centre national de la recherche scientifique.

Olender, M. (1985), 'Aspects de Baubo: textes et contextes antiques', *Revue de l'histoire des religions*, 202: 3–55.

Onians, J. (1979), *Art and Thought in the Hellenistic Age*, London: Thames and Hudson.

Orrells, D. (2005), 'A History of the Critical Theories and Approaches Regarding the Phallus in Antiquity: The Greeks and Modern Masculinity', PhD thesis, University of Cambridge.

Osborne, R. (1998a), *Archaic and Classical Greek Art*, Oxford: Oxford University Press.

Osborne, R. (1998b), 'Sculpted men of Athens: masculinity and power in the field of vision', in L. Foxhall and J. Salmon (eds), *Thinking Men: Masculinity and its Self-Representation in the Classical Tradition*, London: Routledge.

Osborne, R. (2007), 'Sex, agency, and history: the case of Athenian painted pottery', in R. Osborne and J. Tanner (eds), *Art's Agency and Art History*, Malden, MA: Blackwell Publishing.

Osborne, R. and S. Goldhill, eds (1994), *Art and Text in Ancient Greek Culture*, Cambridge: Cambridge University Press.

Østergaard, J. S. (2004), *ClassiColor: Farven in antik Skulptur, Ausst. Kat. Kopenhagen*, Copenhagen: Ny Carlsberg Glyptotek.

Otto, B. K. (2001), *Fools are Everywhere: The Court Jester Around the World*, Chicago: University of Chicago Press.

Padgett, M. (2000), 'The stable hands of Dionysos: satyrs and donkeys as symbols of social marginalization in Attic vase painting', in B. Cohen (ed.), *Not the Classical Ideal. Athens and the Construction of the Other in Greek Art*, Leiden: Brill.

Papademetriou, I-T. (1997), *Aesop as an Archetypal Hero. Studies and Research 39*, Athens: Hellenic Society for Humanistic Studies.

Parker, W. H., ed. (1988), *Priapea: Poems for a Phallic God*, London: Croom Helm.

Parkin, T. (2003), *Old Age in the Roman World: A Cultural and Social History*, Baltimore: Johns Hopkins University Press.

Patterson, C. (1985), 'Not worth the rearing: the causes of infant exposure in ancient Greece', *Transactions and Proceedings of the American Philological Association*, 115: 113–15.

Patterson, O. (1982), *Slavery and Social Death*, Cambridge, Mass.: Harvard University Press.

Peradotto, J. and J. P. Sullivan (1984), *Women in the Ancient World: The Arethusa Papers*, Albany: State University of New York Press.

Perdrizet, P. (1911), *Bronzes Grecs d'Égypte de la Collection Fouquet*, Paris: Bibliothèque d'art et d'archéologie.

Perdrizet, P. (1921), *Les terres-cuites grecques d'Égypte de la Collection Fouquet*, Paris: Berger-Levrault.

Pernice, E. (1904), 'Ererbungen der AntikenSammlungen in Deutschland', *Jahrbuch des Deutschen Archäologischen Instituts*, 19: cols 38–9.

Perry, B. E. (1933), 'The text tradition of the Greek *Life of Aesop*', *Transactions and Proceedings of the American Philological Association*, 64: 198–244.

Perry, B. E. (1936), *Studies in the Text History of the Life and Fables of Aesop, APAM* 7, Haverford, Pa: American Philological Association.

Perry, B. E. (1952), *Aesopica*, Urbana: University of Illinois Press.

Perry, E. (2005), *The Aesthetics of Emulation in the Visual Arts of Ancient Rome*, Cambridge: Cambridge University Press.

Pestilli, L. (2005), 'Disabled bodies: the (mis)representation of the lame in antiquity and their reappearance in early Christian and Medieval art', in A. Hopkins and M. Wyke (eds), *Roman Bodies: Antiquity to the Eighteenth Century*, London: British School at Rome.

Pfisterer-Haas, S. (1994), 'Die bronzenen Zwergentünzer', in G. Hellenkemper Salies, G. Bauchhenss and H.-H. von Prittwitz und Gaffron (eds), *Das Wrack: Der antike Schiffsfund von Mahdia*, Cologne: Rheinland Verlag.

Picard, C. (1958), 'Le nain bossu au coq de Strasbourg', *Gallia*, 26: 83–99.

Pinault, J. R. (1993), 'Women, fat, and fertility: Hippocratic theorizing and treatment', in M. DeForest (ed.), *Woman's Power, Man's Game: Essays on Classical Antiquity in Honor of Joy K. King*, Wauconda, IL: Bolchazy-Carducci.

Pincus, D. (2001), *Small Bronzes in the Renaissance*, New Haven: Yale University Press.

Platner, S. B. and T. Ashby (1929), *A Topographical Dictionary of Ancient Rome*, Oxford: Oxford University Press.

Pollitt, J. J. (1978), 'The impact of Greek art on Rome', *Transactions and Proceedings of the American Philological Association*, 108: 155–74.

Pollitt, J. J. (1986), *Art in the Hellenistic Age*, Cambridge: Cambridge University Press.

Pomeroy, S. B. (1975), *Goddesses, Whores, Wives and Slaves: Women in Classical Antiquity*, New York: Schocken Books.

Porter, J. (1999), *Constructions of the Classical Body*, Ann Arbor: University of Michigan Press.

Potter, P. (1988), *A Short Handbook of Hippocratic Medicine*, Quebec: Editions du Sphinx.

Potter, P., G. Maloney and J. Desautels (1990), *La maladie et les malades dans la Collection hippocratique: Actes du VIe Colloque international hippocratique*, Quebec: Editions du Sphinx.

Potter, T. and C. Wells, eds (1985), 'A Republican healing-sanctuary at Ponte di Nona near Rome and the Classical tradition of votive medicine', *Journal of the British Archaeological Association*, 138: 23–47.

Potts, A. (1994), *Flesh and the Ideal. Winckelmann and the Origins of Art History*, New Haven: Yale University Press.

Prudhommeau, G. (1965), *La danse Grecque antique*, Paris: Editions du Centre National de aa Recherche Scientifique.

Raeck, W. (1981), *Zum Barbarenbild in der Kunst Athens im 6. und 5. Jahrhundert v. Chr*, Bonn: Habelt.

Raeder, J. (1983), *Priene, Funde aus einer griechischen Stadt im Berliner Antikenmuseum*, Berlin: Gebr. Mann.

Ramage, N. and A. Ramage, eds (2008), *Roman Art*, Englewood Cliffs, N.J.: Prentice Hall.

Rasmussen, B. B and J. Lund, eds (2002), *The Past, Present and Future: The Collection of Classical and Near Eastern Antiquities the National Museum of Denmark*, Aarhus: University of Aarhus Press.

Reeder, E. D. (1988), *Hellenistic Art in the Walters Art Gallery*, Baltimore: Trustees of the Walters Art Gallery.

Reich, H. (1903), *Der Mimus*, Berlin: Weidmann.

Reinach, S. (1894), *Antiquités nationales: description raisonnée du Musée de Saint-Germain-en-Laye: Bronzes figurés de la Gaule romaine*, Paris: Firmin-Didot et Cie.

Reinach, S. (1920–30), *Répertoire de la Statuaire Grecque et Romaine*, Paris: Ernest Leroux.

Reuterswärd, P. (1960), *Studien zur Polychromie der Plastik: Griechenland und Rom*, Stockholm: Almqvist & Wiksel.

Reynolds, J. M. and K. T. Erim (1982), *Aphrodisias and Rome: Documents from the Excavation of the Theatre at Aphrodisias*, London: Society for the Promotion of Roman Studies.

Reynolds, J. M. and J. B. Ward-Perkins (1952), *The Inscriptions of Roman Tripolitania*, Rome: British School at Rome.

Rice, P. (1982), 'Prehistoric Venuses: Symbols of Motherhood or Womanhood?', *Journal of Anthropological Research*, 37: 402–14.

Richardson, B. E. (1933), *Old Age Among the Ancient Greeks*, Baltimore: Johns Hopkins Press.

Richer, P. (1902), *L'art et la médecine*, Paris: Gaultier, Magnier et Cie.

Richlin, A. (1992), *The Garden of Priapus: Sexuality and Aggression in Roman Humor*, Oxford: Oxford University Press.

Richter, G. M. A. (1913), 'Grotesques and the mime', *American Journal of Archaeology*, 17: 149–56.

Richter, G. M. A. (1966), *The Furniture of the Greeks, Etruscans and Romans*, London: Phaidon.

Richter, G. M. A. (1984), *The Portraits of the Greeks*, abridged and revised by R. R. R. Smith, London: Phaidon.

Ridgway, B. S. (1984), *Roman Copies of Greek Sculpture: The Problem of the Originals*, Ann Arbor: University of Michigan Press.

Robert, L. (1948), 'Épigrammes du Bas-Empire', *Hellenica*, 4: 1–151.

Robertson, M. (1987), *Greek, Etruscan, and Roman Vases in the Lady Lever Art Gallery, Port Sunlight*, Liverpool: Liverpool University Press.

Rosa, P. (1873), *Relazione tecnica sulle scoperte archeologiche della città e provincia di Roma negli anni 1871–1872*, Rome: Regia Tipografia.

Rose, M. (1997a), 'Constructions of physical disability in the ancient Greek world: the community concept', in D. T. Mitchell and S. L. Snyder (eds), *The Body and Physical Difference: Discourses of Disability*, Ann Arbor: University of Michigan Press.

Rose, M. (1997b), 'Deaf and dumb in Ancient Greece', in L. Davis (ed.), *The Disability Studies Reader*, New York: Routledge.

Rose, M. (1997c), 'Let there be a law that no deformed child shall be reared: the cultural context of deformity in the ancient Greek world', *Ancient History Bulletin*, 10: 79–92.

Rose, M. (1998), 'Women and physical disability in ancient Greece', *The Ancient World*, 29.1: 3–9.

Rose, M. (2003), *The Staff of Oedipus. Transforming Disability in Ancient Greece*, Ann Arbor: University of Michigan Press.

Rose, M. (2006), 'History of disability: ancient west', in G. L. Albrecht (ed.), *Encyclopedia of Disability*, Thousand Oaks: Sage.

Roschach, E. (1865), *Musées de Toulouse. Antiquités: musée des Augustins, Objets d'art: Musée Saint-Raymond, Toulouse*, Viguier: Ernest Roschach.

Ruffer, A. (1910), 'On dwarfs and other deformed persons', *Bulletin de la Société royale d'archéologie d'Alexandrie*, 13: 1–17.

Rumscheid, F. (1998), *Priene: A Guide to the 'Pompeii of Asia Minor'*, trans. R. Blümel, Istanbul: Ege Yayınları.

Rumscheid, F. (2006), *Die figürlichen Terrakotten von Priene: Fundkontexte, Ikonographie und Funktion in Wohnhäusern und Heiligtümern im Licht antiker Parallelbefunde*, Wiesbaden: Reichert.

Russel, P. (1998), 'The Palaeolithic mother-goddess: fact or fiction?', in K. Hays-Gilpin and D. S. Whitley (eds), *Reader in Gender Archaeology*, London: Routledge.

Sacken, E. von (1871), *Die antiken Bronzen des K.K. Münz- und Antiken-Cabinetes in Wien*, Vienna: Braumüller.

Säflund, G. (1963), *Aphrodite Kallipygos*, Stockholm: Almqvist & Winksell.

Sambon, L. (1895), 'Notes on ancient medicine', *British Medical Journal*, 27: 217–20.

Sande, S. (1995), 'An old hag and her sisters', *Symbolae Osloenses*, 52: 30–53.

Savignoni, L. (1901), 'Roma. Nuove scoperte nella città e nel suburbio', *Notizie degli scavi di antichità*, 6: 248–53.

Schefold, K. (1943), *Die Bildnisse der antiken Dichter, Redner und Denker*, Basel: B. Schwabe.

Schneegans, H. (1894), *Geschichte der grotesken Satire*, Strasbourg: K.J. Trübner.

Scobie, A. (1986), 'Slums, sanitation and mortality in the Roman world', *Klio: Beiträge zur alten Geschichte*, 68: 399–43.

Séchan, L. (1930), *Le danse Greque antique*, Paris: E. de Boccard.

Seligmann, S. (1922), *Die Zauberkraft des Auges und das Berufen: ein Kapitel aus der Geschichte des Aberglaubens*, Hamburg: Couvreur.

Shapiro, H. A. (1984), 'Notes on Greek dwarfs', *American Journal of Archaeology*, 88: 391.

Sieveking, J. (1930), *Bronzen, Terrakotten, Vasen der Sammlung Loeb*, Munich: A. Buchholz.

Slane, K. W. and M. W. Dickie. (1993), 'A Knidian phallic vase from Corinth', *Hesperia*, 62.4: 483–505.

Slater, W. J. (1991), *Dining in a Classical Context*, Ann Arbor: University of Michigan Press.

Smith, R. R. R. (1991), *Hellenistic Sculpture: A Handbook*, London: Thames and Hudson.

Snowden, Jr, F. (1970), *Blacks in Antiquity. Ethiopians in the Greco-Roman Experience*, Cambridge, MA: Belknap Press of Harvard University Press.

Snowden, Jr, F. (1976), 'Iconographical evidence on the black populations in Greco-Roman antiquity', in J. Vercoutter and J. Devisse (eds), *The Image of the Black in Western Art*, vol. 1, Cambridge, MA: Belknap Press of Harvard University Press.

Snowden, Jr, F. (1978), 'Blacks in antiquity through the eyes of Greek and Roman artists (summary)', in *Afrique Noire et Monde Méditerranéen dans l'Antiquité*, Dakar: Nouvelles Editions africaines.

Snowden, Jr, F. (1983), *Before Color Prejudice: The Ancient View of Blacks*, Cambridge, MA: Harvard University Press.

Snowden, Jr, F. (1996), 'Bernal's "Blacks" and the Afrocentrists', in M. R. Lefkowitz and G. MacLean Rogers (eds), *Black Athena Revisited*, Chapel Hill: University of North Carolina Press.

Snowden, Jr, F. (2001), 'Attitudes toward blacks in the Greek and Roman world: misinterpretations of the evidence', in E. M. Yamauchi (ed.), *Africa and Africans in Antiquity*, East Lansing: Michigan State University Press.

Spinazzola, V. (1953), *Pompei alla luce degli scavi nuovi di Via dell'Abbondanza*, Rome: Libreria dello Stato.

Spivey, N. (1996), *Understanding Greek Sculpture: Ancient Meanings, Modern Readings*, London: Thames & Hudson.

Squire, M. (2011), *The Art of the Body: Antiquity and its Legacy*, London: I.B. Tauris.

Stackelberg, K. T. von (2009), *The Roman Garden: Space, Sense, and Society*, London: Routledge.

Stevenson, W. E. (1975), 'The Pathological Grotesque Representations in Greek and Roman Art', PhD thesis, University of Pennsylvania.

Stewart, A. F. (1990), *Greek Sculpture: An Exploration*, New Haven: Yale University Press.

Stewart, A. F. (1997), *Art, Desire and the Body*, Cambridge: Cambridge University Press.

Stewart, P. (1997), 'Fine art and coarse art: the image of Roman Priapus', *Art History*, 20.4: 575–88.

Stewart, S. (1984), *On Longing: Narratives of the Miniature, the Gigantic, the Souvenir, the Collection*, Baltimore: Johns Hopkins University Press.

Stieda, L. (1902), 'Die Infibulation bei den Griechen und den Römern', *Anatomische Hefte*, 19: 232–309.

Stiker, H-J. (1999), *A History of Disability*, trans. W. Sayers, Ann Arbor: University of Michigan Press.

Stillwell, R. (1938), *Antioch on-the-Orontes: 2, The Excavations 1933–1936*, Princeton: Committee by the Department of Art and Archeology of Princeton University.

Stillwell, R. (1941), *Antioch on-the-Orontes: 3, The Excavations 1937–1939*, Princeton: Committee by the Department of Art and Archeology of Princeton University.

Strong, E. (1929), *Art in Ancient Rome*, London: Heinemann.

Tabanelli, M. (1963), *La medicina nel mondo degli Etruschi*, Florence: Olschki.

Thompson, D. B. (1954), 'Three centuries of Hellenistic terracottas', *Hesperia*, 23: 72–107.

Thompson, D. B. (1979), 'A faience fellah', in G. Kopcke and M. B. Moore (eds), *Studies in Classical Art and Archaeology: A Tribute to Peter Heinrich von Blanckenhagen*, Locust Valley, N.J.: J. J. Augustin.

Thompson, L. (1989), *Romans and Blacks*, Norman: University of Oklahoma Press.

Thomson, P. (1972), *The Grotesque*, London: Methuen.

Thomson, R-G. (1996), *Freakery: Cultural Spectacles of the Extraordinary Body*, New York: New York University Press.

Tietze-Conrat, E. (1957), *Dwarfs and Jesters in Art*, London: Phaidon.

Tillyard, E. M. W. (1923), *The Hope Vases: A Catalogue and a Discussion of the Hope Collection of Greek Vases*, Cambridge: Cambridge University Press.

Tobler, T. (1863), *De locis sanctis quae perambulavit Antoninus Martyr circa A.D. 570*, St Gallen: Verlag von Huber und Comp.

Tougher, S. (2002), 'In or out? Origins of court eunuchs', in S. Tougher (ed.), *Eunuchs in Antiquity and Beyond*, London: Classical Press of Wales and Duckworth.

Trentin, L. (2009), 'What's in a hump? Re-examining the hunchback in the villa Albani-Torlonia', *Cambridge Classical Journal*, 55: 130–56.

Trentin, L. (2011), 'Deformity in the Roman imperial court', *Greece and Rome*, 58.2: 195–208.

Trentin, L. (2013a), 'Disability in class and classics: towards a more nuanced understanding of ancient history', *Prandium: The Journal of Historical Studies*, 2.1: 55–8.

Trentin, L. (2013b), 'Exploring visual impairment in ancient Rome', in C. Laes, C. F. Goodey and M. L. Rose (eds), *Disabilities in Roman Antiquity: Disparate Bodies A Capite ad Calcem*, Leiden: Brill.

Tronchin, F. (2011), 'The sculpture of the Casa di Octavius Quartio at Pompeii', in K. Cole, M. Flohr and E. Poehler (eds), *Pompeii: Art, Industry and Infrastructure*, Oxford: Oxbow Books.

Tzeng, S-S. (2004), *Changing Bodies: Concepts and Images of the Body in Western Art*, Taipei: Nan tian shu ju.

Uhlenbrock, J. P. (1990), *The Coroplast's Art: Greek Terracottas of the Hellenistic World*, New Paltz, NY: College Art Gallery, The College at New Paltz, State University of New York.

Van Gulik, H. C. (1940), *Catalogue of the Bronzes in the Allard Pierson Museum*, Amsterdam: N.V. Noord-Hollandsche Uitgevers-Mij.

Vercoutter, J., J. Leclant and F. Snowden (1976), *L'Image du Noir dans l'art occidental* I, Fribourg: Menil Foundation.

Vermeule, C. (1977), *Greek Sculpture and Roman Taste*, Ann Arbor: University of Michigan Press.

Vernant, J.-P. (1982), 'Lameness, tyranny, incest in legend and history', *Arethusa*, 15: 19–38.

Versluys, M. J. (2002), *Aegyptiaca Romana: Nilotic Scenes and the Roman Views of Egypt*, Leiden: Brill.

Visconti, E. Q. (1811), *Iconographie grecque*, vol. I, Paris: P. Didot l'aîne.

Vlahogiannis, N. (1998), 'Disabling bodies', in D. Montserrat (ed.), *Changing Bodies, Changing Meanings: Studies in the Human Body in Antiquity*, London: Routledge.

Vlahogiannis, N. (2005), 'Curing disability', in H. King (ed.), *Health in Antiquity*, London: Routledge.

Wace, A. J. B. (1903–04), 'Grotesques and the evil eye', *Annual of the British School at Athens*, 10: 103–14.

Waldhauer, O. (1946), 'Myron's *Anus Ebria* and the drunken woman in Munich', *American Journal of Archaelology*, 50.2: 241–6.

Walker, S. (1995), *Greek and Roman Portraits*, London: Trustees of the British Museum by British Museum Press.

Walters, H. B. (1899), *Catalogue of Bronzes, Greek, Roman and Etruscan in the Department of Greek and Roman Antiquities, British Museum*. London: Trustees of the British Museum.

Weber, W. (1914), *Die ägyptisch-griechischen Terrakotten, Königliche Museen zu Berlin: Mitteilungen aus der Ägyptischen Sammlung*, Berlin: K. Curtius.

Welsford, E. (1935), *The Fool: His Social and Literary History*, London: Faber and Faber.

Williams, C. (1999), *Roman Homosexuality: Ideologies of Masculinity in Classical Antiquity*, Oxford: Oxford University Press.

Wiman, I. M. B. (1990), 'Malstria – Malena. Metals and motifs in Etruscan mirror craft', *Studies in Mediterranean Archaeology*, 91.

Winckelmann, J. J. (1987), *Gedanken über die Nachahmung der griechischen Werke in der Malerei und Bildhauerkunst*, trans. E. Heyer and R. C. Norton, La Salle: Open Court.

Winckelmann, J. J. (2006), *Geschichte der Kunst des Altertums*, intr. A. Potts, trans. H. F. Mallgrave, Los Angeles: Getty Research Institute.

Winter, F. (1903), *Die Typen der figürlichen Terrakotten* III, Berlin: W. Spemann.

Wójcik, M. (1989), *Museo Claudio Faina di Orvieto: Ceramica attica a figure nere*, Perugia: Editori umbri associati.

Wrede, H. (1988), 'Die tanzenden Musikanten von Mahdia und der alexandrinische Götter- und Herrscherkult', *Römische Mitteilungen*, 95: 97–114.

Wrede, H. (1991), 'Matronen im Kult des Dionysos. Zur hellenistischen Genreplastik', *Mitteilungen des Deutschen Archäologischen Instituts, Römische Abteilung*, 98: 163–88.

Yacoub, M. (1969), *Musée du Bardo: Musée Antique*, Tunis: Ministère des affaires culturelles.

Yeames, A. H. S. (1907), 'An ivory statuette', *Papers of the British School at Rome*, 4: 279–82.

Yegül, F. (1992), *Baths and Bathing in Classical Antiquity*, New York: Architectural History Foundation.

Zanker, P. (1974), *Klassizistische Statuen: Studien zur Veränderung des Kunstgeschmacks in der römischen Kaiserzeit*, Mainz am Rhein: P. von Zabern.

Zanker, P. (1995), *The Mask of Socrates. The Image of the Intellectual in Antiquity*, trans. A. Shapiro, Berkeley: University of California Press.

Zanker, G. (2004), *Modes of Viewing in Hellenistic Poetry and Art*, Madison: University of Wisconsin Press.

Zimmer, G. (1982), *Antike Werkstattbilder, Bilderheft der Staatlichen Museen Preussischer Kulturbesitz* 42, Berlin: G. Man.

Illustration Credits

As this is a book about *looking*, images have been included whenever possible. I am grateful to all of the museums and galleries that provided images free of charge (as indicated below); likewise I am enormously grateful to the Faculty of Arts at Wilfrid Laurier University for providing generous funding to support all other reproduction costs. While every effort has been made to contact copyright-holders of images, in the event of any error or oversight the author and publishers will rectify these at the earliest opportunity and provide due accreditation for any future edition.

Illustrations

Frontispiece: © The Trustees of the British Museum, London

Fig. 1. © The Metropolitan Museum of Art / Art Resource, NY

Fig. 2. © 2015 Museum of Fine Arts, Boston

Fig. 3. © Bardo National Museum, Tunis [Photos after Pfisterer-Haas 1994: pls 16–18]

Fig. 4. © Staatliche Museen zu Berlin, Antikensammlung, Inv.-Nr. 8626 [Photo by author]

Fig. 5. © Soprintendenza Archeologica di Pompei [Photo after Tronchin 2011: 39, fig. 2.6]

Fig. 6. Engraving after Visconti (1811) vol. II, pl. 12

Fig. 7. © Musée du Louvre, Paris [Drawing after Reinach 1894: 309, no. 394]

Fig. 8. © Musée du Louvre, Paris [Drawing after Reinach 1894: 309, no. 394]

Fig. 9. © Hatay Arkeoloji Müzesi, Antakya [Photo after Stillwell 1941: pl. 56, no. 120 Panel B]

Fig. 10. © Hatay Arkeoloji Müzesi, Antakya [Photo after Stillwell 1941: pl. 56, no. 121]

Fig. 11. Photo after Stillwell (1941) 25, fig. 27

Fig. 12. © 2015 Museum of Fine Arts, Boston
Fig. 13. © Bikram Rai/WENN.com

Catalogue of hunchbacks

Pl. 2. © Kunsthistorisches Museum, Vienna (without charge)
Pl. 5. © Staat.Antikensammlungen und Glyptothek, München
Pl. 8. © The Metropolitan Museum of Art / Art Resource, NY
Pl. 9. © Walters Art Museum, Baltimore
Pl. 10. After Perdrizet 1911: 163, pl. 107
Pl. 11. © Musée Saint-Raymond, Musée des Antiques de Toulouse (without charge)
Pl. 12. © The Trustees of the British Museum, London
Pl. 13. © Phoenix Ancient Art S.A., Geneva
Pl. 14. © Phoenix Ancient Art S.A., Geneva
Pl. 15. © Staat.Antikensammlungen und Glyptothek, München
Pl. 16. After Carelli 1755–1831: 7: 297–99
Pl. 17. © Hatay Arkeoloji Müzesi, Antakya [Photo after Stillwell 1941: pl. 56, no. 120 Panel A]
Pl. 18. © Staatliche Museen zu Berlin, Antikensammlung, Inv.-Nr. Fr. 2142 a, photo archive (without charge)
Pl. 20. © Musée du Louvre, Paris [Photo after Froehner 1873: 73, pl. 17–18]
Pl. 22. © The Trustees of the British Museum, London
Pl. 23. © Musées de Strasbourg, Musée Archéologique (without charge)
Pl. 24. © Staatliche Museen zu Berlin, Antikensammlung, Inv.-Nr. Misc. 8724, photo archive (without charge)
Pl. 25. © Musée Saint-Raymond, Musée des Antiques de Toulouse (without charge)
Pl. 27. © Kunsthistorisches Museum, Vienna (without charge)
Pl. 30. © 2015 Museum of Fine Arts, Boston
Pl. 32. © Villa Albani-Torionia, Rome [Photo after Alinari Archives, Florence]
Pl. 33. © Museum für Kunst und Gewerbe, Hamburg
Pl. 34. © Staatliche Museen zu Berlin, Antikensammlung, Inv.-Nr. 30894,1, photo archive (without charge)

Pl. 35. © Wadsworth Atheneum Museum of Art, Hartford, CT. Gift of J. Pierpont Morgan (without charge)
Pl. 36. © RMN-Grand Palais / Art Resource, NY
Pl. 37. © Landesmuseum Württemberg, Stuttgart; foto: P. Frankenstein
Pl. 40. © The Trustees of the British Museum, London
Pl. 41. After Gerhard (1965), vol. IV, p. 186, plate 141.1
Pl. 44. © Staatliche Museen zu Berlin, Antikensammlung, Inv.-Nr. Misc. 8756, foto: Jürgen Liepe (without charge)
Pl. 45. After Richer 1902: 177, fig. 109
Pl. 46. © Fine Arts Museums of San Francisco, Museum purchase, M. H. de Young Endowment Fund
Pl. 48. After Perdrizet 1911: 59, pl. 28
Pl. 50. © Musée Saint-Raymond, Musée des Antiques de Toulouse (without charge)
Pl. 52. © 2015 Museum of Fine Arts, Boston
Pl. 55. National Archaeological Museum, Athens © Hellenic Ministry of Culture and Tourism /Archaeological Receipts Fund (without charge)

Index

This is not an *Index Locorum*, but names of ancient authors are here listed.

CPSIA information can be obtained
at www.ICGtesting.com
Printed in the USA
LVOW10s1613070217
523494LV00003B/110/P

9 781350 019140